WHEN
Less
IS MORE

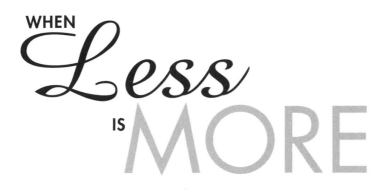

WHEN *Less* IS MORE

THE COMPLETE GUIDE FOR
WOMEN CONSIDERING
BREAST REDUCTION SURGERY

BETHANNE SNODGRASS,
M.D., FACS

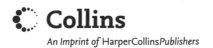

Collins
An Imprint of HarperCollinsPublishers

HarperCollins books may be purchased for educational, business, or sales promotional use. For information, please write: Special Markets Department, HarperCollins Publishers, 10 East 53rd Street, New York, NY 10022.

FIRST EDITION

Designed by Nancy Singer Olaguera/ISPN Publishing Services

Illustrations by R. E. Schneider

Printed on acid-free paper

Library of Congress Cataloging-in-Publication Data

Snodgrass, Bethanne.
    When less is more : the complete guide for women considering breast reduction surgery / Bethanne Snodgrass — 1st ed.
        p. cm.
    Includes bibliographical references and index.
    ISBN-10: 0-06-075874-0   ISBN-13: 978-0-06-075874-5
        1. Reduction mammaplasty—Popular works. 2. Breast—Surgery—Popular works. 3. Surgery, Plastic—Popular works. I. Title.
    RD539.8.S66 2005
    618.1'059—dc22

                                                                    2005040362

05 06 07 08 09 ISPN/RRD 10 9 8 7 6 5 4 3 2 1

To Marianna,

my Sweet Pea

Contents

Acknowledgments

This book has been a labor of love, but it could not have been written without the immeasurable help of so many talented and patient people. I extend my sincerest thanks to the following people for their invaluable contributions: Kris Beard, Wally Chang, Roy Schneider, Art Squires, Jim Stengle, and Hal White. Thanks also go to Bill Ahern, Gary Geiger, Debbie Ibarra, Joanie Koester, Steve Mayo, Jinger Rawski, Delaine Schmitz, Gina Smith, Kelly Kennelly, the pharmacy staff at Flower Hospital, and to Elizabeth Lyon, whose superb book on how to write a successful nonfiction book proposal fulfilled its promise.

I owe a special debt of gratitude to my literary agent, Barbara Lowenstein, for making this book a reality and to the staff at Harper-Collins, most particulary my wonderful editor, Nick Darrell, for so gently but firmly keeping me on the straight and narrow path.

Finally, I am eternally indebted to my family and friends for their unfailing support and encouragement, especially Dolli Darah, Nita Ellis, Monica Malhoit, and Sandy and Louise Mattingly; Mimi, Ari, and Roger; my father, Roger Snodgrass, for being my toughest and most relentless editor; my mother, Mary Ann Snodgrass, for her efforts to teach me the rules of style; my brother-in-law, Steven Peikin, for paving the way and challenging me to follow; and last but not least my sister, Lori Snodgrass Peikin, for far too many things to list, including having the extraordinary good taste to marry Steve.

Foreword

$\mathcal{P}$erhaps no other part of the human body is more synonymous with femininity than the breasts. The social significance attributed to breasts is only reinforced and perpetuated by the media and popular culture. Many times breasts have great significance to a woman's spouse or partner, which places another layer of concern for the woman considering breast reduction surgery and often contributes to her fear and confusion.

Although the medical literature and the Internet are replete with information on the subject, information written for and aimed at the lay audience is almost nonexistent. *When Less Is More* finally bridges this gap. Dr. Snodgrass skillfully dissects the subject of breast reduction and places each component into logical, stepwise, and detailed chapters, keeping the uninitiated in mind. Her language and style are clear and easy to read. Scarcity of professional jargon and medical terminology coupled with clearly illustrated line drawings present each topic in a concise and easily understood format.

In addition, Dr. Snodgrass uniquely includes explanations of the causes and evolution of symptoms associated with mammary hypertrophy, as well as conservative measures to alleviate those symptoms through stretching and exercises.

Dr. Snodgrass includes many details that are often overlooked at the initial consultation and/or during hurried postoperative instructions. Yet all of these details share a common goal: to have a thoroughly informed patient who has been given the tools to make well considered choices and who will face surgery with confidence.

When Less Is More is a must-read for all women considering or facing breast reduciton surgery. Those dealing with this issue owe Dr. Snodgrass a debt of gratitude, for she has eased their way.

Wallace H. J. Chang, M.D.
Professor of Plastic Surgery
Division of Plastic Surgery
University of Washington School of Medicine
Seattle
February 2005

WHEN

Less

IS MORE

Introduction
Can You Get Relief? Yes!

*T*his book is about breast reduction, or reduction mammaplasty, which is surgery to make breasts smaller. If you have ever thought your breasts were too big, this book was written for you. You may be a teenager wearing a baggy shirt to hide your breast size, or you may be a grandmother with deep grooves in your shoulders from your bra straps. You may be a corporate executive, a stay-at-home mom, or you may work two jobs to make ends meet. What you all have in common is that you want to look and feel better. Many of you are dealing with body weight issues, but despite dieting your breast size does not decrease. You want to get relief from your back pain and headaches, you want to be able to buy clothes that fit, and yes, you want to look more attractive. Finally, each of you wants answers to these questions:

- Will a breast reduction really help me?
- Do I have any options besides surgery to help me feel better?
- How do I find a good surgeon?
- Will my insurance pay for the surgery?
- Is the surgery risky?
- If I decide to have surgery, how long will it take for me to be healed and back to my normal routine?
- Is now a good time in my life to have breast reduction surgery?

Whether you are a woman of color concerned about scarring or a busy mom wondering if you will be able to manage your household after surgery, this book will help you. I encourage you to read the entire book before you decide whether you want to have surgery. Then, when you meet your surgeon for the first time, you will already be a well-informed patient. You will get more out of your conversations with your surgeon and, most important, you will feel more confident. You also will find the answers to virtually all of your postoperative questions as you recover and begin to develop your new body image. It is my belief that breast reduction is one of the most effective surgeries available to improve the quality of life for many women, and this book was written to give you the essential information you need before and after surgery.

Twenty years ago I was a plastic surgery resident learning to do the kinds of surgery for which plastic surgeons are famous—face-lifts, rhinoplasties ("nose jobs"), breast augmentations (enlargement with implants)—operations that fall into the category of cosmetic, or aesthetic, surgery. The purpose of these operations is to improve the appearance of "normal" body areas. As a resident I took care of many cosmetic surgery patients as well as hundreds of patients undergoing complex reconstructive procedures to correct deformed, diseased, or injured parts of the body. What really impressed me was a group of patients who fit into both the cosmetic and reconstructive categories— the breast reduction patients. They were some of the happiest patients I had seen.

Plastic surgeons have a wonderful specialty: We are able to help bring happiness to the lives of many people. However, I cannot think of another operation where patients get so much immediate relief as women do after breast reduction. Yes, there are incisions to heal, and yes, reduced breasts take time to resume a natural shape. But this is what I tell my friends who wonder why a woman would want smaller breasts: Imagine living with a sack of flour hanging on a chain around your neck, thinking you will have to wear that load twenty-four hours a day for the rest of your life. Then imagine suddenly realizing that there is a way that you can take the load off and never have to wear it again. Who cannot sense the enormous relief that removing that weight would bring?

Why did I write this book? The simple reason is that more and more women are having breast reduction surgery every year, and there are no books available on the subject for the lay reader. If you have been thinking about breast reduction for a while, you know that before this book was published there was very little information readily available for potential patients. Recently the mass media have been paying more attention to breast reduction, since celebrities such as Queen Latifah, Drew Barrymore, Christina Ricci, Soleil Moon Frye, Mary J. Blige, Roseanne Barr, Patricia Heaton, Loni Anderson, Phyllis Diller, and Nancy Sinatra have all talked about having had breast reduction surgery. Reality television shows such as *Extreme Makeover* have portrayed ordinary people having plastic surgery, including breast reduction. But unless you happen to watch one of the more educational programs featuring breast reduction, you are unlikely to learn very much about the surgery from popular magazines and television. Many women seek information on the Internet because there has been nowhere else to turn. (I always caution patients about the Internet: It is easy to be unnerved by biased and unbalanced comments. Stick with reputable institutional Web sites and avoid chat rooms and other sites where you don't know the source of their "information.") For example, the American Society of Plastic Surgeons Web site has a good summary about breast reduction, and the FDA Web site has a short article on the subject. But comprehensive information in one resource has not been available anywhere, until now.

The incidence of breast reduction surgery has increased 150 percent in the last ten years. When Dr. Robert Goldwyn, a highly esteemed and now retired plastic surgeon, published his textbook *Reduction Mammaplasty* in 1990, he noted in the preface that ". . . reduction mammaplasty continues to be an operation frequently requested and performed. In 1988, an estimated 40,000 were done in the United States." That seemed like a very large number at the end of the 1980s, yet fifteen years later the numbers were still skyrocketing. In 2002, over 100,000 women had breast reduction surgery, and if my practice is any indication, every year three times as many women make appointments with plastic surgeons to get information about the surgery. Breast reduction has become one of the ten most commonly performed major plastic surgical procedures and is performed as often as face-lift surgery.

The main purpose of breast reduction surgery is to relieve symptoms of back, neck, and shoulder pain. Most women having the surgery—which generally removes between four and ten pounds of breast tissue, the equivalent of one or two sacks of flour—experience considerable relief of their symptoms, and one study showed that 98 percent of the breast reduction patients interviewed would recommend the surgery to others. If you are considering breast reduction surgery, you have probably found this to be a difficult decision to make. You aren't alone: Most women say that they chose surgery only after thinking about it for years. Many times, women are reluctant to discuss their complaints with their male family physicians for fear that either they won't be taken seriously or they will merely be told to lose weight. Often these women have additional problems that they don't even realize are related to their breast weight. Here are some of my patients' stories:

❈ Marla came to see me when she couldn't push the sweeper because of back pain. "And it just breaks my heart not to be able to lift my three-year-old grandson," she said. She wore a 36D bra in high school, but after having children her bra size ballooned to 38FF. In the recovery room after breast reduction surgery, she told me, "I feel like an elephant has been lifted off my chest!" Within weeks she was standing up straight, doing housework without pain, and playing freely with her grandchildren. The first thing she said to me at her checkup was, "I wish I had done this years ago!"

❈ "I'm going to have to look for a new job," moaned Keisha, a twenty-six-year-old office worker. She developed large breasts in junior high, and now she is miserable every night after working at a computer all day. I could see the deep grooves in her shoulders, and I explained how her headaches were also probably related to her breast size. She told me that she had been working hard to lose weight, but her breasts weren't getting any smaller. "I tried wearing two bras to aerobics, but I just couldn't take the bouncing, so I quit the class. Buying clothes is a nightmare. Shirts that fit my chest hang off my fingertips! I always have to buy tops two sizes bigger than bottoms. And the guys at work—forget it! Not one of them has looked me in the eye yet."

Rebecca is fifty-one years old, has been large-breasted all her life, and has a cousin with breast cancer. Rebecca tries to stay healthy by watching her diet and exercising, but she has chronic pain in her neck and shoulders from her breast weight. She told me, "I had a mammogram last month, and the radiologist couldn't see all of my breast tissue on the film. So I went back for more X-rays, but he still called the test 'suboptimal.' I came to see you because my family doctor thinks I should consider having breast reduction surgery."

Women with heavy breasts usually suffer for years before seeking help. This book offers you relief by providing you with the information and resources you need to help you feel and look better. The chapters take you in sequence through each stage of decision-making, research, preparation for surgery, the surgery itself, and the entire postoperative period. Terms that may be new to you are in boldface type and are explained in the text and in the glossary at the end of the book.

Chapter 1

The First Step
Will Breast Reduction Surgery Help Me?

It is not easy to think about having surgery on your breasts. American culture is obsessed with breasts. They have become the standard-bearers for femininity. Even as female celebrities' bodies have become thinner, their hips and thighs liposuctioned to look lean and more masculine, their breasts have steadily enlarged. These redesigned bodies are a far cry from the voluptuous nudes of Rubens or even the curvaceous forms of the 1950s' movie bombshells. Yet, as many naturally large-breasted women will confirm, more is not always better. Not every woman wants her breasts to be the center of attention or to enter a room well ahead of the rest of her body. Large breasts can feel like a millstone around a woman's neck, and even large breast augmentation implants weigh less than what most breast reduction patients have removed. Celebrities with surgically enhanced breasts are in the business of selling sex, but ordinary women with oversized breasts often get unwanted sexual attention, both spoken and unspoken. Even worse, their breast size keeps them from living normal lives. In general, the most common problems that cause women to seek breast reduction surgery are back, neck, and shoulder pain; chronic skin-crease irritation; shoulder grooving; and limitations of physical activities. Other reasons that women seek surgery are a significant difference in size between the breasts (breast asymmetry); breast size out of proportion to body size; breast sagging; and self-consciousness or psychological distress due to excessive breast prominence.

Medical research has shown that the more severe a woman's symptoms are, the more likely she is to benefit from breast reduction surgery. Symptoms are more important than breast size in predicting how much benefit a woman will experience from surgery. One study showed that women with pain from heavy breasts ranked living with their symptoms equal to living with chronic medical conditions like low back pain, knee arthritis, moderate chest pain from heart disease, and kidney transplant. Breast reduction surgery has also been shown to improve the lives of women who suffer from heavy breasts by allowing them to resume many routine activities that they had given up because of their symptoms.

In this chapter I will help you analyze your own situation. What kind of symptoms and physical changes do you have that may be caused by your breast size? What medical conditions do you have that might be causing or contributing to your symptoms? Do you want your breasts to be "lifted" but stay the same size? Are there any reasons why you should not have breast reduction surgery?

Throughout this chapter you will see words in boldface type that are the major symptoms and physical changes that insurers look for when evaluating requests for coverage of breast reduction surgery.

SYMPTOMS

❈ Nichole sat on my exam table and told me about her neck and shoulder pain. "They don't carry bras in my size at the store, so I have to order them. It is such a hassle if they don't fit right and have to be sent back. This bra cost $80 and my shoulders still hurt, especially at the end of the day! I get headaches, and some days they are so bad that I just have to sit or lie down until they are bearable. My fingers go numb at night if I sleep on my side, but I hate sleeping on my back." Even so, Nichole wasn't sure what to do. "Do you think a breast reduction would help me?" she asked.

Many women have pain every day that they do not realize is a direct result of their breast weight. I have a series of questions that I ask my breast reduction patients at their first consultation, and almost every patient looks at me with surprise when I ask about a symptom that she never dreamed was related to her large breasts. Once you understand your anatomy you will be able to make a list of your own symptoms.

A woman with large breasts has to support her breast weight with her spine, shoulders, and all the muscles attached to those structures (Figs. 1–1a and b). Your unique anatomy plays a big role in how much breast weight you can handle without symptoms. Your spine is designed to keep your body standing up straight. Actually, your spine is built with natural curves, but the curves complement each other so that your center of gravity ideally is located on a straight line from your ear canal to your ankle. The muscles attached to your spine maintain your posture in its proper alignment. Heavy breasts throw off the alignment of your spine by forcing your neck and shoulders forward

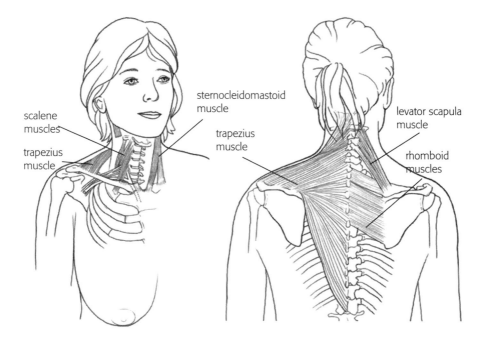

Figure 1-1a Musculoskeletal structures that support breast weight (front)

Figure 1-1b Musculoskeletal structures that support breast weight (back)

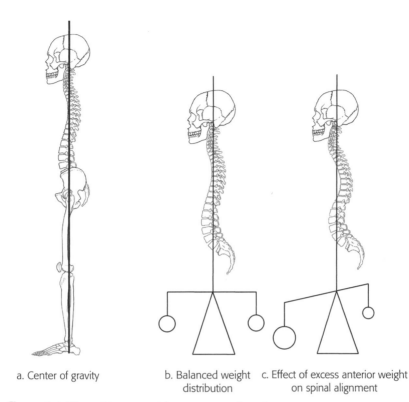

a. Center of gravity   b. Balanced weight   c. Effect of excess anterior weight
                                distribution   on spinal alignment

Figure 1-2 Effect of breast weight on center of gravity

(Figs. 1–2a, b, and c). This changes your center of gravity and puts tremendous strain on your neck muscles. You feel tired more easily, and over time you are more likely to develop bone spurs on your spine that can lead to chronic **neck pain**.

Long-standing neck strain from breast weight can also cause **headaches**. Headaches in the back of your head (occipital headaches) are a common symptom of heavy breasts and result from pressure on nerves that run from the base of your skull up the back of your head. Many women experience relief of these and other kinds of headaches, including frontal headaches and migraines, after breast reduction surgery.

The weight of heavy breasts also affects the position of your upper and middle (thoracic) spines and your shoulder blades (scapulae). Excessive misalignment of these structures puts strain on the attached muscles and ligaments. The shoulder blades roll forward and cause poor posture. Over time these effects cause **shoulder pain**, especially under the bra straps, and **mid-** and **upper back pain**. The pain makes sitting upright difficult, which aggravates your poor posture. Women with a significant difference in breast size (asymmetry) may have greater shoulder and back pain on one side compared with the other.

If you have cared for small children, you know how heavy even the smallest infant feels after carrying him or her around for a few hours. Have you carried a baby in a front pack or a backpack? If you have done both, do you remember which was more comfortable? Someone actually studied the forces exerted on the body with these two carrying methods and discovered that carrying extra weight up front requires more work from the spinal and abdominal muscles than does carrying the same amount of weight on the back. Very large-breasted women suffer more by carrying all that weight on their chests than they would if they could carry those pounds in some other way.

Because your body needs to stay upright in order to walk, any significant change in your center of gravity related to misalignment of your neck, chest, or shoulder area requires compensation by your lower (lumbar) spine. This can cause **lower back pain**, especially if you already have lumbar disc problems.

Regardless of what type of bra a large-breasted woman wears, the weight and size of her breasts can cause irritation of the skin under all parts of the bra. This can lead to occasional or continual **skin breakdown** and **rashes**. Skin breakdown is a particular problem in areas where there is constant skin-to-skin contact and sweating, such as underneath and between the breasts. Rashes that develop in skin creases are called intertrigo, and yeast and bacterial infections may develop if a woman is not vigilant about preventing and treating excessive moisture and early signs of irritation (see Chapter 6).

Heavy breasts put strain on your collarbones (clavicles) and pull on your chest skin. Some women get stretch marks (striae, pronounced "stry'-ee") in the upper chest and breast skin. Many women complain of upper **chest pain** and **breast pain** while exercising or even at rest:

❋ Nancy was telling me about her symptoms when she stopped talking for a minute. Then she went on with a wry smile, "It's embarrassing to admit this, but sometimes, when no one is looking, I just rest my breasts on the table in front of me, just to get a minute of relief for my chest and shoulders."

Forward rotation of your shoulder blades from breast weight and pressure from a tight bra create narrow tunnels under the muscles and ribs at the base of your neck on each side, approximately where your shoulders, neck, and armpits meet. The large nerve trunks that eventually become the ulnar nerves (important nerves to the hands) pass through these tunnels and are often compressed in large-breasted women. Compression of the ulnar nerves causes **arm pain** and **numbness and tingling of the little fingers.** Some women complain of more widespread arm and hand pain, numbness, or tingling.

Many large-breasted women complain that they have **trouble getting to sleep comfortably**. They cannot sleep on their stomachs because of the bulk of their breasts. They cannot sleep on their backs because their breasts shift upward and make them feel as though they are suffocating. If they sleep on their sides, they have to arrange extra pillows to support their breast weight:

※ Over the years I have learned to ask the right questions. Sara rolled her eyes when I asked if she wore her bra to bed. "Are you kidding? I *never* go without a bra, except to take a shower. I sleep in a sports bra. My shoulders kill me from the straps, but it's worse without the support."

Some women complain of **shortness of breath**, especially with exercise, that they blame on their breast size. Think of the weight of your breasts as acting like a lever that makes your chest work harder to expand when you inhale. Breast reduction surgery has been shown to improve chest movement and lung function.

A major problem for large-breasted women that doesn't get enough attention is simply that big breasts get in the way. Most of my patients laugh when they tell me these stories, but the problems aren't funny:

Janet: "Last week I had an important last-minute lunch appointment with a client, and I was frantic. Every blouse in my closet had some kind of food stain on the front of it. When I sit down to eat, my breasts stick out so far I can't even get close to my food. I always try to be the first one at a restaurant meeting so I can pick the table. There is no way I can fit into a booth without my chest ending up literally on my plate."

Sharon: "I was offered a different job at the factory, which I really wanted because it was a sit-down job. I thought it would help my back. But you have to sit at a bench to put small metal parts together, and it's hard for me to see over my chest. If I lean over more it really bothers my back."

Shawna: "I've been playing pool since I was a kid, and I love to be in tournaments. But *these* [she points to her chest] are ruining my game!"

Pam: "I have a summer job at an ice cream shop, but half the time I crush the cones with my chest while I'm trying to scoop up the ice cream. It is so embarrassing I just want to die."

Donna: "It's hard to get a good night's sleep when every time I roll over in bed I have to pick my boobs up and carry them with me."

PHYSICAL EFFECTS

Women with heavy breasts develop predictable physical changes, some of which may be permanent. It is common to have more than one of the following physical signs: **poor posture** and **rounded shoulders** from the effects on the spine, shoulder blades, and muscles, as discussed above; **muscle stiffness** in the neck and shoulders; infected skin creases (**intertrigo**); and **shoulder grooving** with **skin discoloration**. Back and shoulder **muscles are weakened**, not strengthened, in a heavy-breasted woman because her shifted center of gravity puts her back muscles at a mechanical disadvantage. If a woman has already been evaluated by another doctor for her neck pain, she may have had **X-rays showing arthritic changes, including bone spurs.**

Shoulder grooving is the result of years of pressure from bra straps. Brassieres are designed to support the breasts, but in order to support heavy breasts, a bra has to be built almost like a corset. Support comes mainly from underwires, sidewall reinforcement, and shoulder straps. The better-constructed bras have wide, padded straps, but many women buy less expensive bras that fit tightly. (See Chapter 3 for more on buying bras.) A woman who wears a bra that is too tight will find the straps and underwires digging into her shoulders and ribs, and she will eventually develop permanent, discolored grooves in her skin that may crust or bleed:

❉ I usually talk to a new patient before she changes into a paper gown for the physical exam. I asked Anna if she had any pain or indentations of her shoulders where her bra straps ride. "Indentations? You mean the ruts? Oooh, yeah. Those have been getting deeper since high school."

All of these physical changes and their related symptoms progress as women get older. Once a woman passes menopause, her breast size will decrease as the functional tissues in the breast recede. However, very large-breasted women have a tremendous excess of breast skin, and extra skin does not go away after menopause. If anything, skin may sag more and put increasing strain on weakened muscles and on joints and bones susceptible to arthritis and osteoporosis.

More than breast volume may contribute to chest prominence in some women. The distance around your chest (the number part of your bra size, also called chest circumference) increases in women for two reasons: (1) weight gain, in which extra skin and fat develop along the sides of the chest and back, and (2) pregnancy, which causes flaring of the lower ribs. Breast reduction surgery does not correct rib flaring and usually does not include removal of substantial amounts of chest skin and fat that are not part of the breasts. Therefore, after surgery you may wear the same bra size (e.g., 42) but with a smaller cup (42C instead of 42EEE).

Some women have **other medical conditions** that predispose them to the pain from excessive breast weight. These conditions include arthritis and related conditions; fibromyalgia; spinal disc problems, especially in the neck (cervical) and low back (lumbar); a history of fracture or other injury to the collarbone (clavicle) or shoulder; shoulder muscle and joint problems, such as rotator cuff tears; thoracic outlet syndrome, in which nerves and blood vessels are pinched where the armpit, neck, and first rib come together; and other nerve compression problems, such as carpal tunnel syndrome. These conditions can be either the main cause of a woman's symptoms or can be aggravated by her breast weight. If the woman's symptoms are not typical for macromastia (heavy breasts), other causes, including those listed above, should be considered. In this situation your plastic surgeon may refer you to your family doctor or to another specialist for further evaluation. In any case I always counsel potential patients that not every one of their symptoms may resolve or improve after breast reduction surgery.

PSYCHOLOGICAL ISSUES

It would be bad enough if you lived alone on a desert island and had to contend with your oversized breasts, but society adds insult to injury by judging you based on your breast prominence. Your personal issues with your breasts are inevitably intertwined with the demands and judgments of family members, friends, classmates, co-workers, and even complete strangers.

How each woman judges her breasts is influenced by four critical factors in her life: (1) her childhood development and the attitudes of her family members toward the breasts of her mother and other female relatives; (2) the adolescent experiences that helped form her adult sexual identity; (3) the attitudes of the significant people in her life (spouse, children, parents) toward her breasts and toward the idea of her having breast reduction surgery; and (4) the meaning of breasts in the context of the larger society in which she lives, which includes the pressures she may feel to look or behave in a certain way in order to lead the life that she wants to lead.

Psychological concerns can become especially pressing when large breasts are accompanied by severe asymmetry, either developmental (i.e., becomes evident during adolescence) or acquired (for example, after cancer surgery on one breast).

Childhood

From the time of infancy we internalize good or bad feelings about breasts, depending upon our experiences with nurturing and suckling. These feelings develop in both girl and boy infants, whether breastfed or bottle-fed. Since an infant cannot distinguish between what is "me" and what is "Mom," feelings about the breast are processed as feelings about self and are incorporated into the core of the infant's rapidly evolving sense of self. Therefore, the idea of breast reduction surgery for yourself or for a loved one can feel like a threat to the foundations of your personality.

As children grow up they learn attitudes about breasts from the adults around them. A girl's view of her body is formed by her mother's view of her own body, her father's view of her mother's body, and both parents' attitudes toward the child's body. If a girl hears her father make comments, positive or negative, about his wife's breasts, the child will internalize a certain attitude about her own breasts as they develop. If, as is often the case, her breasts are not like her mother's, she may have trouble accepting them as desirable or attractive to herself or to men. A woman with these feelings who wants a breast reduction may have very intense and specific core ideals about how she wishes her breasts to look, and this can lead to disappointment after surgery if she is unaware of or unable to communicate these desires to her surgeon.

Adolescence

The view that a young girl forms of her body, and of her breasts in particular, persists well into adulthood and may in fact last for life. Adolescence, however, may have the most profound effect on a woman's attitude toward her breasts, especially if she matures early. Large-breasted women who say that they were overly endowed even before they had children often report that they were also among the first girls in grade school to develop breasts. Many such girls never become completely comfortable about their bodies, even as adults. Both young girls and adult women suffer from poor self-esteem when they are constantly bombarded with rude or insensitive comments from others. Teenagers suffer the comments of both male and female classmates, and young women have to contend with a predictable array of inappropriate male behavior. My own mother is a well-endowed woman in her seventies, and to this day she remembers with some resentment the way that the boys would snicker when she walked into her junior high school auditorium. Girls with large breasts often become shy and self-conscious around their peers. Their female classmates may express envy, and boys may stare, whisper, and make obscene remarks. Both female and male peers may interpret the mere existence of large breasts as a sexual come-on, even though their owner may have no such intentions. Girls resort to all kinds of behavior to deemphasize their breasts. They start to slouch in junior high school, trying to conceal their breast size, and pick clothes that camouflage their anatomy. They avoid drawing attention to themselves and may refuse to stand up in front of an audience, even in the classroom, or to participate in activities like swimming. They avoid any situation where they have to undress in front of others. They may overeat in an attempt to balance their body proportions by gaining weight. Others may purge in the hope that weight loss will reduce their breast size. All of these behaviors predictably lead to adult problems with posture and weight control, and tend to result in some degree of social isolation.

Family Support

The significant others in a woman's life can support or sabotage her efforts toward change, especially when she is contemplating something as significant as breast reduction surgery. Some family members worry about the general anesthesia. Others worry that they won't be able to function without their wife/daughter/mother for the few weeks required for full recovery. Others may be jealous or threatened that their mother/daughter is having surgery on a body part that has strong symbolic significance in their relationship. (For ideas on how to get your loved ones on board, see Chapter 6.)

PARENTS

Most teenage girls who see a plastic surgeon to discuss breast reduction really want to have the surgery, and in the vast majority of cases their mothers accompany them and support them. However, the relationship between a teenage girl and her mother can be prickly, to say the least, and the surgeon needs to understand the dynamic of this crucial relationship before considering the daughter for breast reduction surgery. In particular, the surgeon should look for evidence of what psychologists call competition, separation anxiety, and vicarious fulfillment. A competitive mother may resent her daughter's desire to become more attractive, for fear that her daughter will outshine her. She may put up all kinds of roadblocks or downplay her daughter's symptoms. By the same token, a competitive mother may encourage her daughter to reduce her buxom appearance and thereby become less of a threat to the mother. Another mother may be having trouble with separation from her daughter. She and her daughter may both be large-breasted, and the mother may fear that by reducing her breasts, her daughter is severing a strong bond of similarity and resemblance between them. "Things will never be the same," the mother may think. This attitude may surface even if the daughter has reached adulthood. Sometimes the daughter herself feels hostility toward her mother for not letting go and seeks out breast reduction surgery as a way to establish her independence. I have also seen this happen when the daughter and mother had very different body types:

❧ One morning I was scheduled to perform breast reduction surgery on a young woman, and when I arrived at the hospital I was intercepted by the nurse who was assigned to my patient. "Your patient is very upset and wants to go home," she warned me. I couldn't imagine what had happened. I had seen the patient, a twenty-year-old single woman, twice in the office and had not noticed any signs of indecision or unusual anxiety. She had come alone both times, even though it is common for young women to bring their mothers to the consultation visits. Even so, our discussions had not suggested any potentially difficult social issues. When I entered her cubicle in the preoperative area, however, the problem became instantly clear. Sitting with the patient was her mother, a thin, small-breasted woman whom I had never met. The mother was very angry. In front of the patient she started to grill me: Why was I encouraging her daughter to have a breast reduction? All the girl has is a weight problem. She (the mother) was absolutely against the surgery and had been telling her daughter for years to lose weight. And on and on. Needless to say, the patient was furious, but she was also in tears and was unable to stand up to her mother. The mother would not allow me to explain the problems her daughter was having and why I felt a breast reduction would help her. Finally, I insisted that the mother leave the room so that I could speak with my patient in private. In the end the mother won. The patient decided to leave without having the operation that she so desperately wanted. All of a sudden I had a new perspective on her consultation visits and instantly understood why she had come to them alone. I never saw her again and have often wondered if she ever managed to break free of her mother's emotional stranglehold.

Finally, in the case of vicarious fulfillment, a mother who has suffered for years with large breasts but who, for whatever reason, has never sought breast reduction, may push her well-endowed daughter to have the surgery, even though the daughter may not be ready psychologically or symptomatically. This mother may say, "I don't want her to suffer the way I have all these years."

Fathers can be supportive or resistant to the idea of breast reduction surgery for their daughters. Unfortunately, fathers are less likely to accompany daughters to the surgeon's office and therefore tend to be less well informed about the surgery, its risks, and its benefits. Often, initially neutral or resistant fathers will become very supportive once this "information gap" is closed. Most fathers simply want what is best for their daughters. Some men, however, persist in believing that a girl is sacrificing her femininity or sexual attractiveness—her "assets"—if she reduces her breast size. In this situation every effort should be made to bring the father to the office so that the surgeon can have a frank and informative discussion with him.

SPOUSE/PARTNER

The typical husband is supportive of his wife's decision to have breast reduction surgery, at least in theory. How well he ultimately copes with the changes in her body depends on how emotionally attached he is to her breasts. Men often have a deep-seated bond with the maternal, nurturing aspects of their wives' breasts and may be threatened by an anticipated loss of this nurturing component of the relationship. By the same token, some men attach strong sexual significance to breasts, especially large breasts. In either case the man in a woman's life may need to be reassured that she will not be flat-chested after the surgery. Men often need more technical details explained to them in order to feel comfortable about the surgery. (Read more on spouse and partner issues in Chapter 11.)

Not every partner is supportive. In *Reduction Mammaplasty*, Dr. Goldwyn relates a poignant story about a woman in her late fifties who sought a breast reduction on the one-year anniversary of her husband's death. It seems that in life he had forbidden her to have the surgery. Even after his death it took her a year to assert her independence.

Most men are tremendously helpful in the postoperative period. Others are not willing to take on "nursing" chores or to provide the emotional support that a woman needs during that time. Others refuse to take time off work or to pick up the extra housework or child care during the woman's recovery period.

Rhonda (crying in my office two weeks after her breast reduction surgery): "I'm trying to follow your instructions and take it easy, but we have two little kids and my husband acts like I should be doing everything by now. He wouldn't do anything around the house after the first week, and he thinks I'm faking it when I tell him I'm sore. My mother came to help but could only stay for three days, and there isn't anybody else I can ask for help."

A woman will do herself a great service if she realistically assesses ahead of time the level of support she can expect from her spouse. (See Chapter 6 for advice on advance planning.)

CHILDREN

Young children should not be involved in the decision-making process for surgery, nor should they be given any details about the operation.

However, they do need appropriate advance preparation. (See Chapter 6 for advice on this issue.)

Social Support

Breasts have always played a powerful symbolic role in human culture, as demonstrated by artifacts that have been discovered, dating from 20,000 B.C. Ever since Paleolithic times, breasts have been celebrated as symbols of fertility and nurturing. Modern-day Americans, however, are obsessed with the erotic aspects of breasts, almost to the exclusion of other parts of the female anatomy. For some women, especially celebrities, acquiring bigger breasts is a goal unto itself, regardless of how disproportionate those breasts may appear. Big breasts shout SEXY FEMALE.

However, you may feel differently. Having carried your large breasts around since early adolescence, you may wish that the world paid less attention to your chest and more to who you are. You may feel that your breasts are sexier to others than they are to you, or maybe that they aren't sexy at all. Still, in the face of all this breast mania, you are not exactly racing to have a breast reduction. This decision is likely one that you have been thinking about for a long time.

How do others really perceive women with big breasts? In many different ways, it seems. Most women are aware of perfect strangers taking notice of a part of their bodies that they may not desire to advertise, and this notice is manifested by everything from staring to outright sexual advances. Sometimes acquaintances and even family members will make comments about a woman's breasts, and at best this can sour a woman's trust in her social relationships. Far worse, when a relative or family friend makes a sexual comment about or touches a young girl's breasts, a line has been unacceptably crossed.

The feeling that some large-breasted women have that they are discriminated against has been supported by the results of academic studies. Women with large breasts may be assumed to be less intelligent or less competent. They may be considered immoral or immodest in segments of society that do not encourage overt sexual display. Women who sense these reactions in others come to resent their breasts.

Some women become preoccupied with their breast size, which can progress to dysfunctional eating patterns. Numerous women have admitted to keeping their weight higher than they would like into order to camouflage or reduce the relative prominence of their breasts and thus discourage unwanted sexual attention. When this behavior develops in a young woman, it establishes bad eating habits that may persist well into adulthood. In some young women, these eating behaviors evolve into pathological eating disorders. A young woman may mistakenly think that her developmental breast enlargement is the result of too much fat in her breasts, and she may develop eating patterns that are consistent with anorexia/bulimia nervosa. In carefully selected cases, breast reduction can be extremely helpful for these women (see Chapter 11).

Some women consider their breasts to be obstacles and handicaps. Others hate their breasts and are disgusted by them. They do not see them as sexual in any way, but rather as a deformity that cannot be hidden. (Some women use their large breasts as a barrier to keep others away and to avoid sexual attention. For these women, reduction of breast size can lead to feelings of vulnerability—see Chapter 8.) Other women try to act as though their breasts don't exist. We all manage to get through doorways and in and out of cars without getting too banged up, because we have learned how tall and wide we are, and our brain helps our body negotiate our daily obstacles. Yet one researcher tells the story of a woman who played poker every week and always managed to knock over the pile of chips with her chest. The researcher theorizes that the woman just did not want to acknowledge how large her breasts were and that they belonged to her.

Similarly, some women are so resentful of their breasts that they subconsciously consider them to be the cause of all of their psychological pain. This "transfer of responsibility" is psychologically dangerous because it prevents the woman from addressing other weaknesses in her personality and developing strengths that will help her cope with life's difficulties.

Different women will have different psychological issues. If you recognize yourself in any of those you read about here, be sure to talk to your surgeon frankly. For example, some women reject their sexual identity as including breasts and literally want to be flat-chested, which in essence means having mastectomies. Some surgeons may not pick up on sexual identity conflicts, and you will not be a happy patient if you are not frank about your motivations. Expect your surgeon to recommend counseling before considering surgery in this situation. Transsexualism is a well-recognized although uncommon phenomenon, and in carefully selected patients, gender reassignment surgeries may be appropriate in the context of a coordinated program of medical and psychiatric management.

Another potential patient at psychological risk is the occasional woman who expects breast reduction surgery to be the solution to all of her life's problems. (This unrealistic motivation is encountered less commonly in breast reduction patients than it is in women contemplating purely aesthetic surgery.) Breast reduction surgery can be tremendously beneficial, but it is not a panacea.

Medical Support

Most women do not investigate breast reduction surgery without first talking to their regular doctors. In fact, an insurance company often requires a woman to go through her primary-care physician "gatekeeper" in order to get a referral to a plastic surgeon. Unfortunately, some primary-care physicians are uninformed about the problems that large-breasted women have. Some women have reported that their family doctors or gynecologists (usually, but not always, male) have discouraged them from having breast reduction surgery, warning them that they will be scarred or distorted or will no longer be attractive to men. I also know women who have been reluctant to bring up the subject of breast reduction with their male doctors, fearful that their complaints will be dismissed or they will be given useless advice (e.g., lose weight). Unfortunately, a few doctors just don't get it. Many physicians do get it, however, especially if they have other patients or family members who have benefited from breast reduction surgery.

LIFESTYLE CHANGES

The symptoms and physical changes of excessive breast weight force many women to change their lifestyles. Most large-breasted women avoid excessive physical activity. Exercise is difficult. Some women, particularly those who are also overweight, have trouble doing even water exercises because their increased body fat causes them to float.

Almost without exception, large-breasted women do not run. Most cannot participate in sports or aerobics, and those who do participate often wear two or three bras for support and to reduce painful bouncing:

Leanne: "I used to be very active. I loved to water-ski, play volleyball, you name it. I always participated in the 10K runs in the spring. I wore two sports bras, then three. After a while it just wasn't worth it. The shoulder and back pain afterward ruined the fun of participating in the event."

More severely symptomatic women have trouble walking long distances. Housework becomes a particular burden, and many women give up doing the heavier chores. Women with young children say how hard it is to lift the toddlers, or how they wish they could participate more in the older children's activities:

Tamara: "I love taking my three children to the playground, but I cannot run after them because my breasts bounce and hurt. Now my back is bothering me so much that I can't pick them up very easily if they fall. This has gotten worse with each baby. This really scares me. If I feel this bad when I'm only twenty-four, what is it going to be like when I am thirty-four? Or forty-four?"

Some women even choose not to nurse their infants because of the logistical difficulties and because they are truly afraid their huge breasts will smother the baby. Some fear that nursing will make their already large breasts even bigger:

Monique: "I always thought I'd have a big family, but after my son was born my breasts got huge. I was so afraid they would get even bigger I stopped nursing him after two weeks. But they never got smaller, and I decided that was it—only one baby for me. He's seventeen now, and I wish I had more kids, but I didn't dare."

Buying clothing can be a nightmare. Bras are essential, even though some women take them off the minute they get home, just to give their shoulders some relief. Bras larger than a DD or DDD cup or wider than 44 or 46 inches often have to be purchased from specialty stores or ordered from catalogs (see Chapter 3) and may be more expensive than off-the-rack bras. Tops are a worse problem. Knits are too revealing. Long-sleeved shirts and jackets that fit across the chest hang off the fingertips. Shopping for a two-piece outfit is an exercise in frustration, since big-breasted women almost always need a different size on the top than on the bottom. Bathing suits present an unwelcome challenge for the same reason.

> *Becka:* "I have a part-time job serving the public, and I have to wear a uniform. I can't get one that fits right, and it is very embarrassing. Most people don't say anything, but they always seem to be staring at me."

Some women have to cut back on their hobbies because of their symptoms. It is always disheartening to hear that a woman has had to give up playing the piano, gardening, or horseback riding because of symptoms related to her breast size, thus depriving her of a way to relax and relieve stress.

Many women report limiting their social activities because of embarrassment or because their symptoms prevent them from participating. This leads to social isolation and depression:

> *Jolene:* "I pretty much stay home anymore. I can't walk very far before my back starts to hurt, and it's embarrassing—I feel like people are staring at my chest everywhere I go. It's hard to keep the house picked up, so we almost never have company."

> *Nina:* "Whenever I go on a date I wear a sweatshirt or keep my coat on the whole time. I feel like the guy must only be thinking about my chest."

ECONOMIC EFFECTS

Women with significant symptoms that are due to heavy breasts are less productive. They limit their activities because of pain and therefore are less fit. They tire more easily and are less likely to take on new challenges. In the workplace this may translate into an employee who is more susceptible to job-related injury and therefore may need more time off from work. A woman looking for employment will reject certain jobs if she feels she is not physically up to its requirements (for example, being on her feet or bending over a worktable for eight hours):

> *Hailey:* "My husband and I always had an agreement that after our kids were in school I would go back and finish my training to be an occupational therapist. I only have a few more hours left to finish. But now I don't know if I can do the job. My breasts are so big that I know they are going to get in the way when I work with patients."

FAILURE OF OTHER TREATMENTS

Women with symptoms from heavy breasts usually try every alternative to surgery that they can think of. Women with mild symptoms may get some relief with **medications, physical therapy**, or better **bras**, but more severely affected women will experience little or no improvement in their symptoms until their breast weight is reduced. So what about **weight loss**? It doesn't work.

Let's face it: Some women with large breasts are overweight. The reasons are genetic, metabolic, dietary, and lifestyle, just as they are for all of us. Sometimes the reason is psychological. I have had more than one patient admit to keeping on twenty or thirty extra pounds just to make the rest of her body more proportionate to her breast size. This extra weight mainly goes to her hips, thighs, and abdomen rather than to her breasts. Many people—including women, doctors, employers, and insurance company representatives—think that a woman has large breasts *because* she is overweight and that all she has to do in order to make her breasts smaller and to relieve her symptoms is to lose weight. *There is no scientific evidence to support this belief or to justify recommending weight loss as an effective method of reducing breast size.* In particular, there is no evidence whatsoever that weight loss is an effective treatment for the symptoms due to heavy breasts. On the other hand, there is plenty of evidence that (1) both overweight and normal-weight women can be large-breasted and can have symptoms related to their breast weight, and that (2) virtually all women, overweight or not, who are candidates for breast reduction surgery for the purpose of relieving symptoms, are likely to benefit from the surgery.

OTHER QUESTIONS THAT YOU MIGHT HAVE

Why Do My 40DD Breasts Hurt My Back but My Best Friend's Don't Bother Her?

We all know large-breasted women who do not seem to be particularly bothered by their breast size, so why are you suffering so much? There are many reasons.

First, no two women are put together exactly the same way. Many people have what are called hypermobile joints, which means that there is more "play" in their range of joint motion. These women (and men) are much more susceptible to the effects of gravity and muscle-overloading imbalances than are people with tighter joint structures. Physical therapists are very familiar with this problem and know that these patients are a particular challenge. A large-breasted woman with hypermobile joints is much more likely to be symptomatic from her breast weight than is a woman with "normal" joint range of motion.

Second, your lifestyle and job requirements play a big role in determining your posture and the way you use your muscles. A woman who sits at a desk or bench, works at a computer, reads, sews, or performs any other activities that involve leaning forward and using her arms and hands more or less at chest or waist level suffers the effects of gravity on her neck and shoulders. The forward position of her head while engaged in these activities and the inevitable rounding of her shoulders strain the muscles that support her head and neck. Some muscles shorten and spasm while others lengthen and weaken, and eventually the changes in the woman's posture become permanent. In contrast, a woman who works as a hairdresser, painter, wallpaperer, or in other jobs that cause her to strengthen rather than weaken muscles in her shoulders and neck may have fewer symptoms related to her breast size.

Third, it is possible that 40DD is *not* your proper bra size. Bra size can be misleading. It is widely known that few women wear their proper bra size, and bra sizes themselves vary tremendously from manufacturer to manufacturer and from style to style even within the same brand. Large-breasted women are notorious for keeping their bras for so long that the bras have stretched out to accommodate breast volume well beyond that for which they were intended.

Fourth, the cultural significance of large breasts in a woman's family and social environment may play somewhat of a role in how comfortable she feels with her breast size. If large breasts are considered a social asset, a woman may be less likely to contemplate making hers smaller despite significant physical symptoms.

Can't I Just Get Rid of the Droopiness Without Going Smaller?

For some women the sagging is the issue, rather than the breast weight. All women experience some degree of sagging of their breasts after weight loss, pregnancy, menopause, or simply as the unavoidable effect of gravity over time. The extent to which this happens depends as much on genetics—your inherited skin type—as on anything else. A surgical procedure that moves the nipple to a higher position on the chest wall and removes excess skin without removing very much breast volume is called a **mastopexy**, or breast lift. Most candidates for mastopexy have few if any physical symptoms related to their breasts, and insurance companies consider this procedure cosmetic surgery. Some mastopexy procedures are similar in design to breast reduction surgery. More information on mastopexy is provided in Chapters 7 and 11.

Is Breast Reduction Surgery Dangerous?

Breast reduction is basically a skin operation and has a very low risk of serious complications. Most women who undergo it are happy with their results and would choose to do it all over again or recommend it to a friend. Naturally, as with any operation, there are risks. Chapters 9 and 10 review in detail the expected results and the potential complications of breast reduction surgery. You should familiarize yourself with these issues before deciding whether to have surgery. Your surgeon also will discuss risks and complications with you, and during that conversation you should ask about any additional concerns that you have.

Can I Afford to Have This Operation?

Even if you have health insurance, you may have trouble getting breast reduction surgery covered (see Chapter 4). If you have mainly psychological or cosmetic concerns and few physical symptoms, your insurance almost certainly will not cover the surgery. If you do not wear at least a D-cup bra, you are less likely to have significant physical symptoms from your breast weight or to get insurance approval. If you are willing to pay for surgery yourself, Chapter 4 includes tips on how to get the most for your money.

When you are considering the financial impact of having surgery, remember that you will be limited in your activities for up to six weeks, longer if you develop a complication. This could be expensive if, for example, you are self-employed and can't rely on paid sick time. Chapter 8 covers the typical activity limitations after surgery in more detail.

Who *Shouldn't* Have a Breast Reduction?

There are many reasons why breast reduction surgery might not be appropriate for a particular woman at a particular time. A woman might:

- be at too high a medical risk for surgery or general anesthesia.
- have incompletely evaluated breast disease or other medical problems.
- have symptoms that are entirely or mostly the result of another problem.
- be too small-breasted for a reduction (she may be a candidate for a mastopexy—see above).
- be too psychologically attached to her breasts, which would put her at risk for significant psychological problems after surgery.

- have inadequate family support, which might compromise her recovery or might result in irreparable damage to important relationships.
- be planning major weight loss surgery, in which case deferral of breast reduction might lead to a better final result.
- be unwilling or unable to comply with the surgeon's instructions before and after surgery or to commit to the "downtime" required to maximize the chances for an uncomplicated recovery.
- not want surgery but feels pressured to undergo it.
- be extremely concerned about losing nipple sensitivity or having scars on her breasts.
- be totally committed to breastfeeding future children.
- be young, minimally symptomatic, and planning to get pregnant.

MAKING THE DECISION

No matter how much you may be suffering from neck pain, back pain, or any of the other symptoms discussed in this chapter, you are probably anxious about the idea of having breast surgery. You may worry about the scars or loss of nipple sensation. Perhaps you worry about having a general anesthesia. These fears are completely normal. As women, we claim much of our identity from having breasts, and the loss of a breast from mastectomy, for example, is a devastating trauma for a woman. Breasts represent femininity, nurturing, and sexuality. Yet some women have a love-hate relationship with their breasts. My patients and their friends and family members frequently joke that for every woman who wants to get rid of some of her breast volume, there is a woman standing behind her who would love to have the excess. On the one hand, a woman with oversized breasts would like to go through a day without pain or to wear a bathing suit without embarrassment. On the other hand, the same woman may be fearful about losing part of her identity as a woman. These fears are common and may persist for a while after surgery (see Chapter 8).

The public and the insurance industry like to label plastic surgery operations as either "reconstructive" or "cosmetic." Breast reduction surgery has a foot on each side of the fence, and it is natural that a woman might feel a little schizophrenic about her motivations. The insurers don't help by penalizing women who exhibit even a whiff of the desire to look better. *Of course* you care about how your breasts are going to look after surgery, and there is nothing wrong with wanting to have relief of your symptoms and better-looking breasts at the same time. Also, understand that you will almost certainly have some anxieties and fears after surgery, even if your physical recovery is smooth sailing.

So what should you do? First, read the rest of this book. Second, think about and write down what it is that you really want. Third, talk to women who have had breast reduction surgery. Fourth, talk to a plastic surgeon. I always say, talk is cheap. You can benefit a lot from talking face-to-face with a surgeon, and you do not have to commit to anything until you are ready.

Chapter 2
From AAA to EEE
Why Breast Reduction Surgery Was Invented

*B*reast reduction surgery has been called the ultimate hybrid plastic surgical procedure, since it offers both medical and aesthetic benefits. It wasn't always that way. The earliest breast reduction operations were practically mastectomies, and the results could hardly be called aesthetically pleasing. This chapter will review the history of breast reduction surgery, the current goals of surgery, the various medical terms that are used to describe large breasts, the surgery to reduce them, and the reasons why breasts get too big.

A SHORT HISTORY OF BREAST REDUCTION SURGERY

An operation to treat breast enlargement in men (gynecomastia) was described 1,500 years ago, but there is no clear record of breast reduction surgery performed for a woman prior to 1800. Safe general anesthesia and fluid replacement have been available only during the last century, and major surgery on a female breast risked significant blood loss. The first known breast reduction for a woman was essentially a breast amputation and was performed in the early nineteenth century. For the next one hundred years, an occasional surgeon performed a primitive breast reduction operation. It was not until the twentieth

century, with the evolution of anesthesia, that surgeons started to perform more sophisticated operations that moved the nipple upward and
protected the blood supply to the nipple and breast skin. By midcen-
tury surgeons had a better understanding of the blood supply to the
breast and started to design and refine operations that could strive
more safely to accomplish the current goals of breast reduction:

- to improve symptoms, including back, neck, and shoulder pain;
  headaches; rashes; nerve compression; and poor posture.
- to decrease the volume and weight of breast tissue without endangering the blood or nerve supply to the nipple and remaining breast.
- to remove excess breast skin.
- to elevate the nipple to its proper position in relation to the
  remaining breast tissue and to the opposite breast.
- to create an improved breast shape that will remain stable over time.
- to accomplish the above goals with a minimum of scarring.

A DEFINITION OF TERMS

Scientific terms referring to the breast come from the Greek "mastos"
or the Latin "mamma." The medical terms for overly large breasts are
macromastia and **mammary hypertrophy**. Massive breast enlargement
is called **gigantomastia** and is discussed in Chapter 11.

The medical term for breast reduction surgery is **reduction
mammaplasty**. The operation includes removal of excess skin, fat, and
glandular breast tissue. The areola (pigmented area around the nipple)
is usually made smaller, and the nipple and areola are moved to a
higher position on the chest. The reduced breast tissue is reshaped to
form a smaller mound. As mentioned earlier, a similar operation called
mastopexy is designed primarily to correct breast sagging and removes
minimal breast volume.

WHY BREASTS GET BIG

Humans have remarkably diverse body shapes, and there does not
always seem to be an obvious reason why a particular woman develops
large breasts. The following is a short review of breast development
and the reasons for breast enlargement.

Breasts are specialized skin glands and start to appear very early during the development of a fetus. Breast tissue grows along the milk lines that extend from the armpit to the groin. Most of the tissue in the milk lines disappears before birth except for the area over the pectoral muscles. This area becomes the breast and nipple. Occasionally, more tissue persists as extra (ectopic) breast tissue in the armpit or as an accessory nipple along one of the milk lines.

Breasts are composed of **milk lobules** that form glands similar to sweat glands; **ducts** that drain the glands to the nipple; **connective tissue** (tissue that holds everything together); **fat**; and **skin**. The tissues that make up a large breast are *not* usually abnormal. A large-breasted woman does not necessarily have relatively more gland tissue or more fat tissue than a woman with smaller breasts. Women as a group vary tremendously in the amounts of fat, gland tissue, and skin in their breasts, regardless of breast size.

For the most part, the breast lies over ribs 2 through 6, but breast tissue can be found in the armpit (axilla), upper abdomen (epigastrium), chest muscle (pectoralis), chest skin, and along the edge of the back muscle (latissimus dorsi). The breast has blood supply from three directions and contains a series of small tubes called lymphatics that connect with lymph nodes in the armpit and in the middle of the chest. Breast infections or tumors may cause the lymph nodes to enlarge, which is why your surgeon will examine these areas during your preoperative breast exam. Multiple nerves from three directions provide sensation in the breast and nipple.

The breast is attached to the chest wall (to muscles and to a thick layer over the muscles called fascia) and, by bands called Cooper's ligaments, to the skin. The strength of these attachments varies from woman to woman, and women with loose attachments will show the effects of gravity more severely than will women with tight attachments. No surgical technique has ever been developed that can reliably prevent the effects of gravity on the breast.

Nipple position varies tremendously from woman to woman, and it is very common for the nipples to be asymmetrically positioned on a woman's breasts. Nipples may point straight down, straight forward, toward the armpits, or toward each other.

At birth only the main breast ducts and a small, flat nipple are present. This remains a girl's anatomy until she reaches puberty, when hormones cause fat and connective tissue to increase in her breasts.

The ducts enlarge and lengthen, but the milk-producing lobules of the glands do not develop fully until pregnancy. At that time the lobules expand and divide into smaller compartments called alveoli.

Genetics

Body type is inherited but not always as you might expect. We all know large-breasted women whose sisters and mother wear B cups. Your large breasts may come from your paternal grandmother or from an even more distant relative. By the same token, your daughters may or may not share your body shape and breast size.

Hormones

Breast tissue is affected by nearly every hormone produced by the body. Hormones from the ovaries, adrenal glands, pituitary gland, and brain (hypothalamus) work together to influence breast growth and function beginning before birth and continuing throughout a woman's life. The most important hormone causing breast enlargement is estrogen, which is released by the ovaries. Estrogen triggers growth in breast tissue by attaching to cells at points called estrogen receptors. Women with overly large breasts usually have normal blood levels of estrogen and the normal number of estrogen receptors. Therefore, the main scientific theory explaining excessive breast enlargement is that breast tissue in some women is hypersensitive to estrogen. You might guess that it is the gland tissue in the breast that responds the most to estrogen, but in fact it is the fibrous tissue and fat that are most sensitive to the hormone. The important point here is that breast enlargement for the majority of potential breast reduction patients is due to increases in *hormone-sensitive* breast fat and fibrous tissue and is not due to increased body fat that happens to be in the breast and that can be expected to shrink with weight loss.

The first big change in breast size occurs during puberty. Girls destined to become large-breasted are usually the first in their class to start developing breasts. These girls may have breast buds as early as age eight, and breast development can precede other obvious signs of puberty by as much as two years. Breast enlargement may continue even after a teenage girl reaches her adult height. Dramatic and often painful massive breast enlargement during the hormone stimulation of adolescence is called gigantomastia (see Chapter 11).

Pregnancy causes a woman's breasts to enlarge, and they remain enlarged until lactation ceases. Once a woman stops nursing (or if she doesn't nurse at all), the milk glands and the increased blood flow in her breasts start to shrink. These effects are the result of changes in hormone levels and take six months to a year to be complete. There is tremendous variation among women in the permanent effects of pregnancy and nursing on breast size. A particular woman's final breast size and shape after pregnancy are influenced both by how much her breasts responded to her temporarily elevated hormone levels and by her skin tone. Some women experience permanent breast enlargement that does not respond to weight loss. These women often find that their breast size progressively increases with each pregnancy. Other women's breasts return to approximately their prepregnancy size and shape. Still other women lose much of their original breast fullness, due to shrinkage of the glandular breast tissue. Some of these women have poor skin elasticity and are left with elongated, flat, drooping breasts. Even these women can have significant symptoms related to their breast size, since the excess skin is heavy and does not lessen with weight loss.

By the time a woman reaches the age of thirty-five, her ovarian hormone production starts to drop, and the glandular portions of her breasts start to shrink further. After menopause, when her ovarian hormone production stops completely, her breast ducts and glands degenerate until her breasts are made up almost entirely of skin, fat, and connective tissue.

Hormones taken as medication can cause breast enlargement or can reduce the degree of breast tissue shrinkage that normally occurs during menopause. Both birth control pills (taken for contraception or to regulate the menstrual cycle) and hormone replacement therapy (HRT) for menopausal symptoms can cause breast enlargement.

Obesity

The exact relationship between obesity and breast enlargement is unclear. Obese women do not necessarily have disproportionately oversized breasts, and most heavy women who are also very large-breasted say that weight loss has little effect on their breast size.

Women who gain weight *after* breast reduction surgery usually do not have to move up to a larger bra cup size.

Skin Laxity

The tightness or looseness (laxity) of your skin—that is, skin tone—is a key factor determining your breast shape and size. Skin contains collagen and elastin, two important proteins that determine how well your skin resists gravity and reacts to injury. The quality of your skin proteins is almost entirely genetically determined. In other words, you inherited your skin tone, and you have very little control over how your skin behaves. If your skin proteins are strong and tightly linked together, your skin can return to its original shape even after prolonged stretching. For a woman the ultimate test of skin elasticity is pregnancy. A woman with excellent skin elasticity may show few signs of having been pregnant. She is the one you see with her kids at the pool, and you assume she must be the babysitter. Let's face it: She is the exception. The typical woman completes a pregnancy with the twin gifts of a beautiful baby and extra skin on her breasts and belly. If you have stretch marks, they are an indication that the bonds of your skin collagen and elastic fibers have split. These changes are permanent and, depending on severity, are associated with varying degrees of skin laxity and sagging.

Obesity followed by weight loss has an effect on skin that is similar to the effects of pregnancy, as does the natural aging process. Because skin elasticity varies so much from woman to woman, two women with the same breast volume may have dramatically different breast shapes. The woman with good skin tone may have dense, "up front" breasts, while the woman with poor skin tone will complain that she has to fold her breasts to get them into her bra.

Two factors that permanently damage skin proteins but over which *you do have control* are ultraviolet-light exposure (from natural sunlight or a tanning booth) and smoking.

Who Has Large Breasts?

Women with large, heavy breasts span all socioeconomic categories, most ethnic groups, and all postpubertal ages. Even though weight loss usually does not correct their problems, women with large breasts are frequently overweight. This is not surprising, as obesity is considered to be a constantly worsening epidemic in the United States. The National Institutes of Health (NIH) classifies nearly two-thirds of adult American women as overweight or obese. Nonetheless, there are still significant numbers of women who are not overweight but who have large breasts for the reasons discussed earlier in this chapter.

When Is a Breast Too Big?

Not surprisingly, there is no single or "right" answer to this question. Academic papers have been published about the ideal breast size, stated to be about 275 grams (B or C cup), but the ideal size is surely in the eye of the beholder. To a physician, a woman's breasts are too big when she has significant symptoms or physical signs related to her breast size. Beyond that, it is a woman's perception of her breast size that counts. A woman's breasts may be too big when they cause shoulder pain, when she can't see the food on her plate, when she can't find clothes that fit, when she is embarrassed by their prominence, or when they prevent her from leading a normal life. If a woman is physically active, especially if she is involved in sports, or if she has other medical problems, such as arthritis, she may be more hindered by even moderate breast hypertrophy than is a similar-sized woman with a more sedentary lifestyle.

By no means should every woman who thinks her breasts are too large have breast reduction surgery, but if you *are* considering surgery, it is my goal to educate you about its realities, risks, and benefits.

WHEN IS THE RIGHT TIME TO HAVE BREAST REDUCTION SURGERY?

The typical woman who comes to my office to discuss breast reduction surgery has suffered for years before suspecting that much of her daily pain has been related to her breast size. In some cases her family doctor has been puzzled by the severity of her symptoms in the face of minimal findings on X-rays or blood tests, and may not realize how significant the weight of large breasts can be. In other cases the family doctor has encouraged her to consider breast reduction, but she is having a hard time acknowledging that her breast weight is the source of her problems.

A woman may think about having breast reduction surgery at any point in her adolescent or adult life. A large segment of my breast reduction practice is women between the ages of twenty-five and forty-five who have finished childbearing. I also see plenty of younger women who have never been pregnant but who already have significant symptoms, as well as many older women whose symptoms are worsening as their joints start to ache and muscles gradually weaken.

There is no single "best time" to have a breast reduction, but for most women certain times in life are better than others. A teenager ideally should wait until her breast size has been stable for more than a year. A young woman who is not severely symptomatic and plans to get pregnant soon may want to consider waiting until after her last pregnancy, especially if she has a strong commitment to breastfeeding. A woman who plans to have a gastric bypass for weight reduction will likely develop a significant degree of skin laxity and breast sagging after major weight loss. She will have a nicer breast contour if she delays breast reduction surgery until she has achieved a substantial portion of her intended weight loss. Any woman who has significant medical problems needs to have those problems stabilized through good medical management before considering any elective surgery, including breast reduction. Her other physicians should agree that her breast reduction surgery may be performed without undue risk.

Chapter 3

Choices
Your Alternatives to Surgery

*M*ost breast reduction patients wish that there was a way their breasts could become smaller without surgery. I do not know of another way, but in this chapter I will show you what you can do to help relieve your symptoms, at least temporarily. Unfortunately, no one has been able to come up with any alternative to surgery that predictably and permanently relieves the symptoms of heavy breasts.

FINDING A GOOD BRA

Most women wear bras that do not fit properly, and I find that the typical large-breasted woman has no idea what her correct bra size is. Since bras tend to stretch out over time, and since large bra sizes are harder to find and can be expensive, many women simply squeeze into their old bras for as long they can. When a patient of mine decides that she is ready to proceed with breast reduction surgery, I often recommend that she be professionally measured so that I can report her correct bra size to the insurance company. A sales clerk may measure you if you shop at a department store or a store that sells mainly lingerie, but I recommend that large-breasted women go to a shop that caters to women who wear plus sizes or who have had breast cancer. These shops employ experienced, board-certified fitters, and they stock or can order bras that will fit your needs. Certified fitters are accredited by either the Board for Orthotists/Prosthetists Certification or the American Board for Certification in Orthotics and Prosthetics.

To get a rough idea of your bra size, measure yourself with a tape measure. First, put your bra on and measure the distance around your chest at the level of the crease under your breasts. Be sure that the tape measure stays parallel to the floor and touches your bra all the way around your chest. Do not pull the tape tight and do not measure while inhaling. Write down the measurement in inches. If the number is less than 33, add 4 inches. If the measurement is more than 33, add 3 inches. You now have your bra circumference number. Next, measure your chest again, but this time around the fullest part of your breast. Use that number to find your cup size according to the following table:

Cup Size	Inches
AA	34
A	35
B	36
C	37
D	38
E (or DD)	39
F (or EE or DDD)	40
G (or FF, etc.)	41
H	42
I	43
J	44

Each 1-inch increase in chest diameter across the breasts represents a move up to the next cup size, although commonly the letter representing the smaller cup size will instead be duplicated (DD equals E, DDD equals EE equals F, etc.). Manufacturers may make any bra in a regular or full cup, with the full-cup version fitting a fuller breast.

Never buy a bra without trying it on first. Different styles within the same brand will fit differently. When you put on a bra, be sure that your breasts are centered in the cups. Lean forward and "shake" your chest so that your breasts settle into the cups. Fasten the bra with the middle row of hooks. If the bra feels too tight across your chest, try the next wider size. If your breasts bulge out of the cups, try a bigger cup size. If the cups wrinkle, try a smaller cup size. Turn sideways so that you can see both the front and back of the bra in a mirror. If the bra feels comfortably snug but the back is not level with the front (i.e., the back rides up), lengthen the straps.

Unfortunately, there is no single industry standard for bra sizing, so different brands may fit differently. This is the main reason why you should be professionally measured if you wear anything over a DD cup or if you are considering breast reduction surgery.

What should you look for in a bra? This is what the professionals say:

- **Support**

First and foremost, you need support. If you cannot tolerate under-wires, look for bras made with newer, stiff fabrics that function like an underwire but do not poke or dig into your ribs and skin. These bras are especially helpful for women who have wide breasts or who have fullness along the sides of the chest under the arms. Molded cups are more substantial than nonmolded.

- **Straps**

Straps can be the traditional adjust-in-the front style or the "cami-straps" that slide to the back, but make sure that they are wide and of good-quality material. Straps should *not* stretch. Padded straps are the most comfortable. Make sure that the straps are attached to the back of the bra toward the middle of your back rather than toward your sides (closer to a V shape rather than an H shape, as viewed from the back) or they will tend to slide off your shoulders. If you find a bra that you like in all other respects except for the position of the straps, you or the shop seamstress can detach and reposition them.

- **Wide back**

A wide bra back with multiple hooks distributes the load of your breast weight over a broader area and will keep you more comfortable through the day.

- **Fabric**

Look for a bra that is made of a soft but substantial fabric that feels as if it will help support your breasts. Otherwise, all of your breast weight will be hanging off your shoulders, and all of the pressure from the bra will be on your rib cage. Avoid microfiber, which is very soft but does not provide enough support.

- **Elasticity**

The bra should be built with some horizontal (side to side) but minimal vertical (shoulder to belly) "give" or elasticity. Test the bra by stretching it in both directions.

- **Seams**

Seamless bras are not for you. They simply do not provide enough support for a large breast. Look for bras with fabric-covered seams and hardware.

- **Correct size**

If you are like many large-breasted women, you are overflowing your bra, both at the top and along the sides. If, when you take your clothes off, there are marks on your skin in the shape of your bra, you need a bigger bra. Go to a professional fitter to find the correct size and a quality brand. Then buy three bras—one to wear, one to wash, and one to rest. Your bras will last longer this way. If you decide to shop by catalog or on the Internet, be sure that a professional fitter has measured you first so that you know your exact size, brand, and style before you order. It is a good idea to buy at least your first bra at a local shop so that you can be sure that it is what you want.

Remember, no two bras are the same, so don't assume that the pretty new bra style you just ordered in your size will fit. If you want to order online, be sure to check the return policy in case what you ordered doesn't fit correctly.

- **Brands**

The companies that make bras for department stores or lingerie shops rarely make anything bigger than a DD cup. In order to find a bra that is the correct size and of good quality, you need to visit a shop that sells brands designed for plus-size women. These brands include Goddess and Aviana. Shops that serve women with breast cancer also carry bras made by Camp and Amoena that are designed for mastectomy patients but that can be worn by anyone. These bras look like regular bras but are made of higher-quality materials and workmanship than the average off-the-rack bra.

Queen Latifah has been promoting a brand of bras aimed at "curvaceous" women called Curvation. These bras are available at discount stores, but again you may not find sizes larger than 44DD.

- **Cost**

You should be able to buy a good-quality bra for $40 to $50. You can spend more for style, but don't be fooled by a store clerk who tells you that nothing in your size is available for less than $60 or $70.

- **Sports bras**

If you participate in sports, you need a lot of support, more than is usually present in sports bras. Look for the features mentioned above, especially molded cups and a Y-shaped back. Bras that close in the front tend to have more fabric and thus more support in the back. Also look for breathable fabric and big armholes. Bras with hooks are easier to get on and off than are those without fasteners. Several Web sites sell sports bras for larger women, although you probably won't find many choices if you need more than a DD or DDD cup. Try www.title9sports.com, www.activasports.com, or www.sierrablue.com.

MEDICATIONS

Pain is an almost universal symptom of heavy breasts. If you have pain, your natural response is to try to relieve it. Sometimes changing your posture can make your back feel better. For some women resting their breasts on the table in front of them provides instant relief. Chronic muscle strain can lead to pain in those muscles and associated ligaments and joints, and this type of pain may not be so easily relieved. Some women may experience temporary benefit from medications for these symptoms.

Over-the-Counter Pain Medications

Aspirin, acetaminophen (for example, Tylenol), ibuprofen (for example, Advil, Motrin), and other pain medications sold in supermarkets and drugstores may provide some temporary relief from mild pain symptoms. However, they should be taken according to the directions on the bottle or by a physician's recommendation. All drugs, even those sold over the counter, have risks, especially if taken for long periods. If you find yourself taking the maximum recommended dosage of a nonprescription pain medication every day for weeks, you should discuss your symptoms with your doctor.

Anti-inflammatories

Otherwise known as NSAIDs (nonsteroidal anti-inflammatory drugs), these include prescription-strength ibuprofen and numerous other related drugs that help reduce the inflammation that can cause muscle, ligament, and joint pain. These drugs usually have to be taken for several weeks before the anti-inflammatory effect kicks in. They can have side effects—most commonly stomach upset or even ulcers, and bleeding—and should be taken under a doctor's supervision. Any drug that can increase bleeding should be discontinued at least two weeks before any major surgery (see Chapter 6 for a list of drugs in this category). Anti-inflammatories in the COX-2 inhibitor category (Celebrex, Bextra, and Vioxx) have recently come under increased scrutiny because of an apparent increased risk of heart attack for patients taking high doses of these medications. Check with your doctor or pharmacist if you have questions about any anti-inflammatory medication you may be taking.

Steroid Injections

Women who develop chronic pain in a particular location, such as in the shoulder joint or shoulder muscle (rotator cuff) area, may benefit from referral to a specialist, such as an orthopedic surgeon or a rheumatologist. These doctors are experienced in evaluating and treating joint problems. They may recommend an injection of steroid medication into the inflamed area, which may result in significant long-term pain relief. Steroid injections cannot be repeated indefinitely, however, since excessive amounts of steroids can lead to undesirable thinning of tissues or even rupture of the injected structures.

Muscle Relaxants

Some physicians prescribe muscle relaxants (for example, Flexeril, Norflex, Zanaflex, Soma) for conditions that cause muscle spasms.

Most of these drugs are intended for short-term use after a specific incident or injury that caused the muscle spasms. These drugs are related to antidepressants and affect the brain rather than the muscle directly. They are not intended for treatment of long-standing problems like the chronic strain on muscles, shoulder joints, and the spine experienced by most heavy-breasted women.

Narcotics

Severe pain requiring treatment with narcotics indicates that the patient has another significant problem in addition to heavy breasts. Nonetheless, breast reduction may be of considerable benefit for patients with severe underlying diseases, such as cervical arthritis or spinal disc disease, for which the patient may be taking narcotics.

PHYSICAL THERAPY

If you have a lot of symptoms in your neck, shoulders, and back *and* you have a very disciplined personality *and* you want to avoid surgery, I strongly recommend that you start a program of physical therapy. You will probably need a prescription from your doctor, and you may be required to have a physical examination and undergo testing, such as X-rays or an MRI, before starting therapy. Most important, you should find a therapist who is well trained and experienced in treating neck and shoulder problems. Your therapist will teach you a stretching and strengthening program that you can use at home, and you need to keep in mind that you will have to incorporate this program into your daily routine, lifelong. Even if you do eventually have surgery, you will find that the physical therapy exercises will help counteract the unavoidable effects of gravity and lifestyle that give us all pains in the neck!

The three key elements of a successful physical therapy program for problems related to heavy breasts are: (1) postural retraining, (2) muscle stretching, and (3) muscle strengthening. Other modalities, such as whirlpool, heat or cold applications, and manipulations, can provide temporary relief, but in and of themselves offer no permanent improvement of the underlying muscle imbalances. The following exercises may be helpful but do not take the place of a complete evaluation and treatment plan by a qualified physician and physical therapist. Do not attempt the following exercises if you have any medical or physical contraindications (i.e., health or safety-related reasons why you should not engage in these activities).

Postural Retraining

I always warn my patients: Gravity is not your friend! Gravity is pulling your breasts down, and your breasts are pulling your neck and shoulders forward, even if you are wearing a bra. Meanwhile, your neck is trying to hold up the weight of your head, and the rest of your spine is realigning itself to keep your body from falling over. The best muscles for keeping you properly lined up are getting weaker, and the weaker muscles are working overtime and causing you pain.

You need to break this cycle, and in order to do that you are going to have to literally retrain your brain. You have to fight against the habit of trying to hide your breasts. Here are some exercises that will help:

1. You must learn to think of yourself as *Tall*, whether you are sitting or walking (Fig. 3–1). You must restore the muscle balance in your neck and shoulders, and the first step toward accomplishing this is to become constantly aware of your posture. Get into the habit of checking your posture frequently throughout the day. **Stand tall** when you find yourself slouching. By thinking tall you will automatically roll your shoulders back and start to realign your neck and lower back. **Tuck your chin**, keeping your head straight, until you feel the stretch at the base of your skull. This may not feel good at first, but will improve as you work on the stretching and strengthening exercises. You may hate this exercise because it feels like you are giving yourself a double chin, but you will be amazed at how good this stretch will eventually feel.

2. In order to support your lower back you must **strengthen your abdominal muscles.** I know, I know; you hate crunches. Well, the good news is that they don't work very well anyway, so you don't have to do them. Instead, do the following exercises once or twice a day (Note: If you are doing these maneuvers correctly, they should not cause pain in your back):

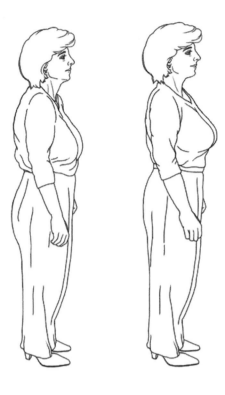

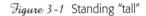

Figure 3-1 Standing "tall"

- Lie on your stomach on the floor (Fig. 3–2). Prop yourself up on your elbows (which should line up directly below your shoulders) and your toes, if possible. If you can't do toes, use your knees instead. Balance in this position and hold for 20 seconds. Rest. Repeat 4 times.

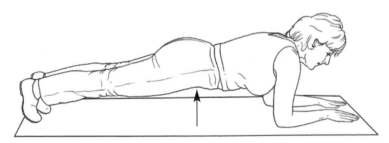

Figure 3-2 Abdominal muscle strengthening, prone

- Lie on your right side (Fig. 3–3). Prop yourself up on your right elbow, which should line up directly below your shoulder. Raise your hips off the floor until your body is in a straight line. Hold this position for 20 seconds. Relax. Repeat 4 times. Do the same exercise lying on your left side.

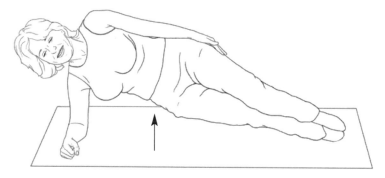

Figure 3-3 Abdominal muscle strengthening, lateral

- Lie on your back with your legs straight if possible. If this is uncomfortable, bend your knees (Fig. 3–4). Flatten the lower part of your back against the floor. Hold for 20 seconds. Relax. Repeat 4 times.

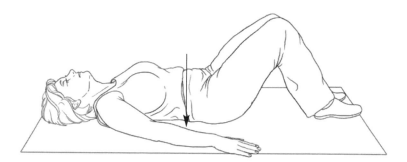

Figure 3-4 Abdominal muscle strengthening, supine

Muscle Stretching

Multiple muscles in your neck and shoulders shorten when your posture is out of alignment. You can feel them as hard, tender cords or lumps. By stretching these muscles and allowing them to return to their proper length you will be able to strengthen other muscles in your back and shoulders that will help support your breast weight.

CHEST MUSCLES

These exercises stretch the **pectoralis major** and **pectoralis minor,** which are two big muscles that extend across your chest.

1. Lie down on your back with a rigid foam roller 6 inches in diameter and 3 feet long under your head and spine lengthwise (Fig. 3–5). (You can order these rollers online for about $20. Try www.performbetter.com.) Your arms should be straight along your sides, with your hands touching the floor. Gradually spread your arms out, trying to position them at right angles to your body (so that you form a T), palms up, and let the weight of your arms stretch your chest muscles. It may take a session or two to form that T.

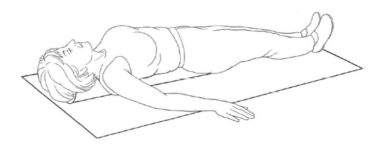

Figure 3-5 Chest muscle stretch with roller

2. Stand just in front of a doorway with your feet together (Fig. 3–6). Stand tall; tighten your abdominal muscles; tuck your chin. (You should not be feeling any new shoulder pain.) Extend your arms out to the sides and position your palms to face the walls or doorway trim. Inch forward until your hands touch the doorway on either side, then lean your body gently forward until you feel the stretch in your chest muscles. Hold this position for 20 seconds. Relax. Raise your arms to

form a V and repeat the stretch. Relax. Repeat the sequence 2 times. Perform this exercise several times a day.

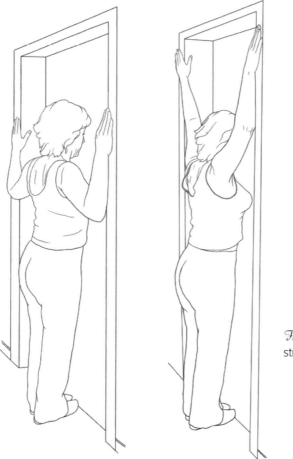

Figure 3-6 Chest muscle stretch, standing

NECK MUSCLES

This exercise stretches the **scalene** muscles, which are deep muscles in the front of your neck:

1. To stretch the right scalenes, rotate your head slowly, about halfway around to the right (Fig. 3–7). With the tips of the fingers on your left hand, push down gently in the hollow behind the center of your right collarbone (this maneuver stabilizes your first rib). Now tilt your head back slightly and tip your left ear toward your

left shoulder. (You may not get your ear very far down for the first day or two.) Hold for 20 seconds. Relax. Repeat 2 times on the same side. Repeat the entire process in mirror image for the left side stretch. Do this sequence several times a day. While doing this stretch, do not push your head down with your hand and do not elevate your shoulders.

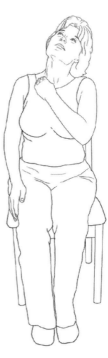

Figure 3-7 Neck muscle stretch

SHOULDER MUSCLES

1. This exercise stretches the **levator scapulae**, a muscle in your back that elevates your shoulder blade:

   • Sit on an armless chair (Fig. 3–8). For the right side stretch, use your right hand to grab the right side of the chair seat (this keeps your right shoulder down and back). Tilt your head forward and turn your chin slightly left. With your left hand pull the back of your head gently toward your left knee. Slowly lean your body to the left and slightly forward, looking toward your left knee, until you feel the stretch in your back just above your right shoulder blade. Hold the stretch for 20 seconds. Relax. Repeat 2 times on the same side. Repeat the entire process in mirror image for the left side stretch. Do this sequence several times a day.

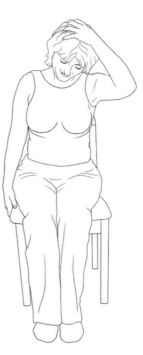

Figure 3-8 Upper back muscle stretch

2. This exercise stretches the upper **trapezius** (the big muscle that runs along the side of your neck to your shoulder) and the **sternocleidomastoid** (a long muscle that runs at an angle from near the bottom of your ear to the middle of your collarbone).

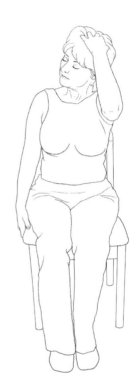

- This is how to do the stretch for these muscles on the *right* side: Sit on a straight-backed armless chair (Fig. 3–9). Rotate your head to the right and tilt it so that your left ear is facing your left shoulder and your chin is pointing toward your right shoulder. Support your head with your left hand. Grab the right side of the chair seat with your right hand and lean your body slightly forward and toward your left knee until you feel the stretch in the *right* side of your neck. You can move your chin from side to side to stretch the two muscles better. You may also press down on your head gently with your left hand to improve the stretch. Hold each stretch for 20 seconds. Relax. Repeat on the same side. Relax. Perform the mirror-image procedure for the left side neck muscles.

Figure 3-9 Shoulder and neck muscle stretch

Muscle Strengthening

Stretching and strengthening exercises are often recommended together to help reestablish muscle balance. Some patients, especially those with joint hypermobility, may need to start stretching and strengthening very slowly in order to avoid destabilizing their joints. Strengthening can be done with isometrics, free weights, Therabands (color-coded stretchy lengths of rubbery material, available wherever physical therapy supplies are sold), or on weight machines.

The muscles that need to be strengthened are in your upper back and shoulder area. They include the **middle and lower portions of the trapezius** muscle and the **rhomboids**. These exercises can be done on the floor, on a bench, or standing. (An acceptable substitute for a workout bench is a large, high footstool or an ottoman.) The key to doing these exercises is to *avoid working the upper trapezius muscle*. The upper trapezius is activated when you elevate your shoulders, so do not hunch your shoulders during these exercises. Look at yourself in the mirror. Look at your bra straps where they cross your collarbone. Just behind the collarbone is a little depression, then a thick band of muscle running from your skull just behind your ear down toward your shoulder joint. This is the upper part of your trapezius muscle. This is also the muscle that begs to be massaged when someone puts his or her hands on the top of your shoulders. The upper trapezius muscle tends to work overtime in patients with shoulder problems and may have trigger points or sometimes feel like it is burning.

FLOOR EXERCISES

Here is how to start strengthening exercises on the floor (preferably on a mat) using isometrics. Isometric exercises are those in which your muscles work against resistance without much shortening. In other words, the muscles tense but the joints to which they are attached do not move. In these exercises you are working against gravity. For each exercise do two or three sets of 10 to 20 repetitions each. Do not rush your repetitions: Slow and steady is more effective. Rest for 30 to 60 seconds between sets.

1. Positioning is everything in this exercise. Lie on your stomach on a mat (Fig. 3–10). Rest your forehead on a small pad, just big enough to keep pressure off your nose while you look straight at the mat. Rest the backs of your hands on your buttocks. Tuck your chin. While doing this exercise, *keep looking straight down at the floor*. Do not look up. Lift your head and shoulders as a unit off the floor. Eventually, try to get your chest off the floor and aim to hold each contraction for 10 to 20 seconds. If you are doing this exercise correctly, you can feel the curve of your cervical spine (neck)

straighten when you tuck your chin. You should also feel the stretch in the deep muscles along your spine, not in the upper trapezius running between the side of your neck and your shoulder.

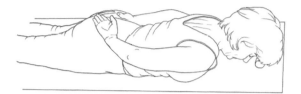

Figure 3-10 Upper back muscle strengthening I

2. While you are in the same position, extend your arms straight along your sides, thumbs toward the floor (Fig. 3–11). Slowly raise your arms off the floor, keeping your elbows straight. Lower and repeat as above.

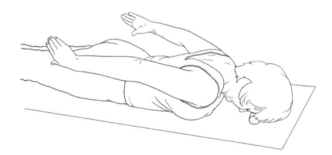

Figure 3-11 Upper back muscle strengthening II

3. Remaining in the same position on the floor, extend your arms along the floor above your head, thumbs up (Fig. 3–12). Keep your elbows straight and slowly raise your arms off the floor. Lower and repeat as above.

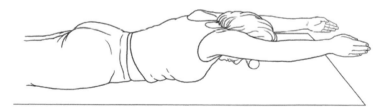

Figure 3-12 Upper back muscle strengthening III

4. In the same position, rotate your arms 90 degrees from your body, keeping thumbs up and elbows straight (Fig. 3–13). Slowly raise your arms off the floor. Lower and repeat as above.

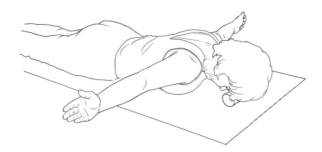

Figure 3-13 Upper back muscle strengthening IV

BENCH EXERCISES

1. You can do all of the floor exercises on a bench using free weights. How much weight? Start low (1 pound per hand) and work up to whatever weight you can manage.

2. Lie on your stomach as in the preceding exercises (Fig. 3–14). Extend your arms at right angles to your body, bend your elbows, and allow your forearms to dangle to the floor. Grip your weights. Roll your shoulders back as though you were trying to touch your shoulder blades together. Relax and repeat as above.

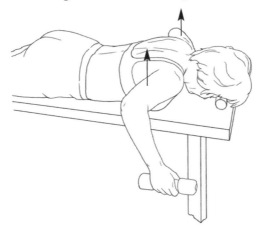

Figure 3-14 Upper back muscle strengthening V

If you can retrain your brain, improve your posture, and strengthen other back muscles, you may be able to reduce the activity of the upper trapezius, which should help your shoulder and neck pain.

WEIGHT LOSS

Plastic surgeons and their breast reduction patients have known for decades that making breasts smaller relieves back and neck pain and many other symptoms, and that weight loss as an alternative treatment does not work. Women who successfully lose weight often find that their pants fit better, their chest diameter is smaller, but their bra cup size is unchanged.

Family doctors and insurance companies do not always understand the lack of correlation between breast size and body weight. A woman who complains to her primary-care physician about her breast size may be given diet advice. Some insurance companies claim that weight loss is a cheaper, safer, and effective treatment alternative to breast reduction surgery. Other insurance companies, if they cover breast reduction at all, may use body weight, body mass index, body surface area, or some combination of these as criteria to determine who should receive coverage. Unfortunately, because these measurements are not accurate indicators of whether surgery is medically appropriate, many women are wrongly disqualified for coverage of breast reduction surgery. As a result, overweight women (who often cannot exercise because of symptoms related to their breast size) are frequently denied coverage of the very operation that will allow them to increase their activity level and lose weight more readily. There has never been any scientific rationale for the use of body weight criteria to assess the "medical necessity" of breast reduction. There are, however, numerous studies showing that weight loss is not an effective treatment for reduction of breast size *or* for relief of symptoms related to heavy breasts.

The fact that no studies have ever shown that weight loss helps relieve the symptoms of heavy breasts was a crucial part of a U.S. District Court decision in 1996. The case involved a plaintiff, who had been denied insurance coverage of breast reduction surgery based on her weight, and her insurance company. The judge found for the plaintiff, stating that there was no medical evidence to justify the insurance company's requirement that the patient lose weight before surgery, whereas there was plenty of medical evidence proving the effectiveness of breast reduction surgery.

Interestingly, we now know from medical studies that not only do both heavy and normal-weight women benefit from breast reduction, but that breast size in breast reduction patients remains stable for years, *regardless of whether the patients gain weight after surgery.*

OTHER TREATMENTS THAT MAY HELP

You may find that some or all of the following treatments (in alphabetical order) help your symptoms in the short term, but none fully address the underlying problems of excess breast weight or muscle imbalances:

- Acupuncture
- Biofeedback
- Chiropractic treatment
- Electrical stimulation
- Massage
- Relaxation techniques
- Yoga

FADS

Women who want a breast lift for strictly cosmetic reasons are usually less accepting of the scars that come with traditional breast reduction surgery. Breast lift without scars is an elusive goal. So far it has been nearly impossible to undo the effects of gravity without removing breast weight and skin. Therefore, physicians are always looking for new solutions. Currently, Botox is all the rage, and a physician recently reported doing breast lifts with Botox. This procedure cannot be expected to have lasting results. My advice regarding the "latest" procedure, whatever it may be, is that any woman should be extremely cautious if encouraged to choose a new and unproven treatment option.

Chapter 4
Confidence
Finding a Surgeon

$\mathcal{B}$reast reduction surgery is a component of all approved plastic surgery training programs and is not part of standard training in any other surgical specialty. This chapter will help you find a plastic surgeon who is right for you. You should be able to get quite a bit of information before you ever meet with a plastic surgeon. Later, your consultation visit will provide you with more knowledge about the surgeon's experience, compassion, and commitment to your well-being.

QUALIFICATIONS

You want your surgeon to have met all of the qualifications to practice plastic surgery and to be in good standing in the community. **Beware!** There are physicians out there performing procedures like breast reduction who are not plastic surgeons and who have had *no formal surgical training*. Be sure to check credentials. The following are universally recognized basic quality standards:

Licensure

All physicians must be licensed by a state medical board in order to practice medicine. Every hospital is supposed to check the status of a physician's license every time the physician reapplies for privileges to bring patients to the hospital, usually every two years. A physician's license can be suspended for failure to complete sufficient continuing education hours or for more serious problems, such as substance abuse. Physicians occasionally lose their medical licenses for serious or repeated offenses. Actions by the state medical board to restrict or revoke a physician's license are a matter of public record.

You can find out whether a physician has an active medical license in your state by contacting the state medical board or by checking its Web site.

Plastic Surgery Specialty Training

Plastic surgeons learn their skills in plastic surgery residency or fellowship programs, which they enter after medical school and only after receiving training in general surgery. Some plastic surgeons have also had training in another specialty, such as otolaryngology (ear, nose, and throat) or dentistry. The plastic surgery segment of a surgeon's training usually takes two or three years, or longer if significant research experience is included. Some plastic surgeons will have spent even more time training in a subspecialty area, such as hand surgery or craniofacial surgery (remodeling the skull and facial bones in babies with birth defects). These plastic surgeons may focus their practices on their subspecialty and may do little if any breast reduction surgery.

Board Certification

Board certification is a voluntary process for physicians. However, a physician's certification by a recognized medical board has become generally accepted not only as a way for patients to assess the physician's basic credentials, but also as a requirement by hospitals, physician groups, and insurance companies for physicians who wish to participate in those organizations.

The major medical specialties in the United States have certification boards that are members of the American Board of Medical Specialties (ABMS). Boards other than the twenty-four boards approved by the ABMS may not have the same standards for physician training and evaluation as do the approved boards. If a physician is board-certified by an ABMS-approved board, it means that he or she has met certain criteria established by peers in the same specialty. These criteria include successful completion of an approved training program in the specialty and a passing score on a certification examination. Surgeons newly out of training may be required to wait a year or more before they are permitted to take the certification examination, and during this period they are generally referred to as "Board Eligible." Board eligibility does not last indefinitely, and if a surgeon fails to complete the requirements for board certification within the allowed time period (usually several years), he or she must complete additional training in order once again to become eligible to take the certification examination.

The **American Board of Plastic Surgery** is an ABMS-approved board and has developed strict standards for its diplomates. It is the only ABMS-recognized board that certifies physicians in plastic surgery on all areas of the body. In order to become certified by the American Board of Plastic Surgery, a physician must graduate from an accredited medical school and must complete a certain number of years in general surgery training followed by plastic surgery training. (The current minimum requirement is three years of general surgery and two years of plastic surgery.) The physician must then pass comprehensive written and oral examinations. Plastic surgery is also among several specialties that now require diplomates certified after 1995 to take a recertification exam every ten years in order to maintain board certification. Within the next few years all ABMS boards, including the American Board of Plastic Surgery, will be shifting to an expanded Maintenance of Certification (MOC) program, which will be mandatory for plastic surgeons receiving their initial board certification in 2007 or later and wishing to maintain their certification. Plastic surgeons who became board-certified prior to 1995 have been "grandfathered in" and are not required to take recertification exams or to participate in the MOC program.

There are many ways that you can determine if a plastic surgeon is certified by the American Board of Plastic Surgery. The American Board of Medical Specialties operates a toll-free phone line (1–866-ASK-ABMS) to verify the certification status of individual physicians. You can also access this information through links on the ABMS Web site at www.abms.org. Certified specialists are listed in *The Official ABMS Directory of Board Certified Medical Specialists*, published by Marquis Who's Who. The ABMS *Directory* can be found in most public libraries, hospital libraries, university libraries, and medical libraries. You can also request the status of a physician's board certification from your county medical society. More information about the American Board of Plastic Surgery can be found on its Web site at www.abplsurg.org.

Society Memberships

Most physicians belong to at least one, and frequently to several, professional societies. The American Medical Association (AMA) is the most well-known medical society, but specialists tend to be more active in societies devoted to their particular field of practice. The American Society of Plastic Surgeons (ASPS) is the largest plastic surgery specialty organization in the world and has over five thousand member surgeons. Like board certification, membership in the ASPS is voluntary, but if your surgeon is a member, he or she has met certain criteria: board certification by the American Board of Plastic Surgery or the Royal College of Physicians and Surgeons in Canada; regular participation in continuing education activities; maintenance of a strict code of ethics; and agreement by the surgeon to perform all surgeries requiring anything more than minor local anesthesia in an accredited, licensed, or Medicare-approved facility. (For more information see the APSP public consumer Web site www.plasticsurgery.org.) Plastic surgeons whose practices include cosmetic surgery may belong to the American Society for Aesthetic Plastic Surgery (ASAPS), which has similar requirements (see www.surgery.org).

Hospital Privileges

Even if a surgeon has an office-based operating room, he or she will have some patients that need to be in the hospital. Find out where the surgeon has privileges to do breast reduction surgery. Avoid a surgeon who does not have privileges to do surgery in any hospital in your area—this likely means there is a problem.

EXPERIENCE

Look for a plastic surgeon with both an interest in and experience with performing breast reduction surgery. It is perfectly acceptable to ask how many breast reductions he or she has performed. Some plastic surgeons do very few breast reductions—for example, one or two a year or even less—because their primary interests are in other areas of the specialty. As with all types of surgery, your surgeon's degree of experience is the best predictor of a good result.

REFERENCES

Assuming that you have identified the plastic surgeons in your community who have satisfactory qualifications and experience doing breast reduction surgery, your best next step in choosing a surgeon is to seek out references from multiple sources:

Other Physicians

One of the best reference sources is another surgeon who has actually worked in the operating room with the plastic surgeon you are considering. Since someone like that may not be available to you, ask your family physician or other physicians you know for a recommendation. If your insurance company requires you to have a referral from your primary-care physician, you are probably being sent to the plastic surgeon with whom your family doctor is most comfortable. Nonetheless, it doesn't hurt to ask your doctor about his or her experience with patients who have had breast reduction or other surgery by the plastic surgeon you plan to see.

Previous or Current Patients

If you know or can arrange to meet someone who has had breast reduction surgery by the surgeon you are considering, you will get a lot of information about that physician. It is helpful to have more than one reference for a surgeon in case you meet someone who seems excessively unhappy or even excessively happy with her results. The surgeon may be able to provide you with the names of patients who would be willing to talk to you about their experiences. During your consultation with the surgeon, ask if there are other breast reduction patients with whom you can talk. Naturally, these will be happy patients selected by the doctor, but that does not mean that they cannot share a lot of helpful information and answer many of your questions, A few words of warning here in case you get a firsthand look at someone else's result: Every woman's body is unique, and your end result cannot be fairly predicted based on that of another patient.

Friends and Family Members

Even though perhaps no one you know personally has had breast reduction surgery, you should still be able to find people who have experience with at least some of the plastic surgeons in your community. Ask around.

APPROVED PROVIDER

Unless you are planning to pay for your surgery out-of-pocket, near the top of your to-do list should be finding out if the plastic surgeon is an approved provider on your insurance plan. If the insurance company requires one, get a referral from your family doctor for evaluation by the plastic surgeon.

THE CONSULTATION

Your first visit with a plastic surgeon will be the most comprehensive. You should leave his or her office armed with information and with a good sense of the doctor's ability to help provide a solution to your problems. The following is a summary of the typical elements of a consultation visit:

Consultation Fee

If your insurance company will not pay for you to see a plastic surgeon, you will have to pay for the consultation visit on the day of your appointment. Less commonly, a plastic surgeon may give free consultations to patients interested in cosmetic surgery, such as breast lift (mastopexy). Ask in advance about the consultation fees.

Complete Medical Evaluation

Now is your opportunity to describe the problems you are having, the length of time they have been troublesome, and your efforts (successful and unsuccessful) to treat them. You may be asked a series of questions to help the surgeon get a complete picture of your situation. Some surgeons ask these questions face-to-face. Others use a medical history form that you will be asked to fill out. Some offices may have a nurse or physician's assistant obtain this information from you. You will be asked about your family history of breast problems; the status of your mammogram testing; and your height, weight, and bra size. It is helpful if you have recently been professionally fitted for a bra so that you know your correct size (see Chapter 3). There are two main reasons for this: (1) Your surgeon will have your correct bra size to state in the letter to the insurance company, and (2) you and the surgeon's staff will know what size sports or surgical bra you will need after surgery. If you decide not to have surgery, you will at least have found a source for buying good bras that fit.

You will be asked for a complete medical history at the time of your first consultation. The history includes all medications that you take, reactions you have had to medications, allergies, current conditions for which you see a doctor, past surgeries, past hospitalizations, and anything else that might affect your health. Be wary of a surgeon who does not request this information. If your health history is extensive, write down the details at home and bring the list with you. Be sure that the surgeon has the name of your primary-care physician. Especially important is any history of the following:

- Current medications, including vitamins; over-the-counter medications; occasional medications; inhalers; topicals; eye drops; nutritional supplements; and herbals
- Use of steroids within the past year
- Current or recent (within six months) use of Accutane

- Drug allergies, intolerances (including to pain medications), and reactions
- Latex allergy
- Allergies to foods, tape, dyes, iodine, or other substances
- Use of tobacco, alcohol, or recreational drugs
- Heart problems, including mitral valve prolapse
- High blood pressure
- Breathing problems or lung disease
- Respiratory infections
- Prior personal or family problems with anesthesia
- Blood clots of any kind
- Diabetes
- Anemia (low hemoglobin or oxygen-carrying capacity)
- Use of blood thinners or any personal or family history of bleeding problems
- Implanted devices or prostheses, such as pacemakers, heart valves, or artificial joints
- Current or recent pregnancy or breastfeeding
- Breast cancer
- Prior breast surgery
- Rashes or infections in or around your breasts, such as in the creases
- Chronic infectious conditions
- Urination or bladder problems
- Recent significant weight loss, stringent dieting, or use of diet pills
- Eating disorders
- Psychological problems or psychiatric treatment or counseling for any reason
- Religious, traditional, ethnic, or cultural practices that may impact your care

Your physical examination will include body areas pertinent to your symptoms and proposed surgery. Your breasts will be examined for size, shape, nipple position, and signs of breast cancer or other breast conditions. If there are any suspicious findings in your breasts or armpits, the surgeon will likely refer you to the appropriate specialist for further evaluation and diagnosis. The surgeon will also look for signs of skin problems, shoulder grooving, postural abnormalities, muscle spasms, and any other signs related to excess breast weight.

The surgeon may take some measurements and will estimate how much weight can be removed from each breast, as well as your ultimate bra cup size. The typical patient goes down two or three cup sizes, less for small reductions and dramatically more for very large reductions. In any case, bra size can only be estimated and never guaranteed. The more important number is the weight estimate, which gives you an idea of how much relief you will experience. Photographs will be taken of your chest and shoulders. These pictures will be sent to the insurance company, along with a letter requesting coverage of your surgery. Some surgeons use patient photographs for teaching or marketing purposes and are required to obtain your consent before doing so.

Discussion

After the examination the surgeon will explain your options, and you should make sure that the surgeon understands your goals for surgery. If, for example, you feel that your nipples are too big now or you fear that your breasts will be too small after surgery, speak up now. You will learn the risks, potential complications, and the anticipated long-term results of breast reduction surgery. You should also be made aware of what specific characteristics you have that may affect the outcome, such as your current breast size and shape, body shape, age, medical conditions, and the condition of your skin. The surgeon will emphasize the extent of scarring that you can expect and the particular risks to your nipples. This is the time to ask about nipple inversion (usually not corrected at the time of surgery because of concerns about blood supply) and reduction of excessively large nipples. If losing nipple sensitivity is a very big concern, you may want to think twice about having the surgery. You will learn what type of anesthesia your surgeon recommends, your options as to the facility at which the surgery will be performed, and your financial obligations. You and the surgeon (plus your spouse or parent, if present) should discuss these options until you feel comfortable with your understanding of them. Make the surgeon aware of any opinions or concerns that you have.

Be sure to tell your surgeon if you have a particular breast size and shape in mind. Your goals in this regard may or may not be realistic, and now is the time to find out. All doctors are under pressure to see more patients these days, and they may not pick up on subtle clues indicating that a patient does not understand some aspect of the proposed treatment.

Do not be shy about getting the information that you need. Read Chapter 7 of this book before you go to your consultation visit so that you understand the basic concepts of breast reduction and the various options for surgery. Come to the consultation prepared with a written list of questions, so that you can listen to the surgeon instead of worrying that you will forget to ask something. At a minimum the following questions should be answered during this discussion:

Will breast reduction surgery help me?

Is this a good time for me to be undergoing this operation?

Are there alternatives to surgery?

Will my insurance pay for the surgery?

Where will the surgery be performed?

What kind of anesthesia will I have?

What are the risks?

What will my breasts look like after surgery?

What complications could I have and how would they be treated?

How much time will I be off work, and how much help will I need?

Am I at any increased risk compared with a typical patient?

Will I need free nipple grafting? (See Chapter 7.)

Will I have much breast fullness after surgery?

Should I consider breast implants? (See Chapter 7.)

You should never feel pressured by the surgeon to undergo surgery. This is your decision to make. The surgeon should gladly answer any questions you have about his or her professional qualifications, experience with breast reduction surgery, or financial issues related to the surgery.

If you do decide to have surgery, some surgeons offer, and I strongly recommend that you take, the option of a second consultation visit prior to your surgery date so that, if necessary, the surgery can be reviewed and all of your remaining questions can be answered. This also gives you a second opportunity to speak with the surgeon face-to-face prior to the day of surgery.

Planning Your Surgery

If you have decided to pursue surgery, the planning process can be started during your consultation visit. If you are going to be financially responsible for the surgery, payment details will be worked out. If not, and assuming that you are generally healthy, you and the surgeon will wait for a response from the insurance company as to whether your surgery will be covered. In either case you may be asked to sign a financial responsibility form. But if you have any medical problems or take any medications that might increase your risk of complications, your surgeon may require more input from your primary-care doctor or other physicians. For example, you may be asked to have a complete physical examination, heart evaluation, or lung testing. If you will need to stop or adjust medications, such as insulin or blood thinners, the appropriate specialist will be asked to provide the necessary orders. See Chapter 6 for detailed information on how to get ready for surgery. If you have evidence of skin irritation or infection, the surgeon will recommend specific treatment. You may receive prescriptions for an iron supplement or antibiotics. Be sure to take these medications only as prescribed.

Financial Obligations

Do not leave your surgeon's office without discussing who is going to pay for the surgery, including follow-up care and the treatment of any complications that might develop. Chapter 5 discusses this issue in detail.

Facility Options

If you decide to have surgery, you want assurances that you will be cared for in a safe environment by well-trained professionals. Your facility options may include a hospital, an outpatient surgery center, or an office surgery suite. Most breast reductions are performed in a hospital-based facility. Financial concerns often influence what type of facility is chosen (see Chapter 5).

Regardless of where your surgeon recommends that you have the surgery, it should be performed in a facility that meets at least one of the three following criteria: (1) accreditation by a national or state-recognized accrediting agency/organization, such as the American Association for Accreditation of Ambulatory Surgery Facilities (AAAASF), the Accreditation Association for Ambulatory Health Care (AAAHC), or the Joint Commission on Accreditation of Healthcare Organizations (JCAHO); (2) certification to participate in the Medicare program under Title XVIII; (3) licensure by the state in which the facility operates. These requirements ensure that appropriate staffing and equipment are available to monitor you safely and to deal with potential complications or emergency situations. If your surgeon cannot provide you with this information about the recommended facility, you can ask for a phone number for the facility so that you can make your own inquiries. You can also find out about a facility's accreditation status by contacting the AAAASF at 1-888-545-5222 or www.aaaasf.org; the AAAHC at 1-847-853-6060 or www.aaahc.org; and the JCAHO at 1-630-792-5005 or www.jcaho.org.

Find out who will be administering your anesthesia or sedation. Any planned anesthesia should be administered by skilled, licensed personnel acting under the direction of an anesthesiologist or the operating surgeon.

If your surgery is scheduled for the surgeon's office, find out the qualifications and number of medical personnel who will be in the operating suite during surgery. You should be assured that you will receive individual monitoring by skilled, licensed personnel who are trained in advanced cardiac life support (ACLS). If the facility does not have overnight capabilities, there must be a transfer plan for patients who are not ready to go home by the end of the day.

If the facility does have twenty-four-hour capabilities and there is a possibility that you will be kept overnight, you should expect to receive around-the-clock care and monitoring by two or more skilled and licensed staff members, at least one of whom is trained in ACLS. Again, there must be a transfer plan in case you require hospitalization.

If you have a significant medical condition such as heart or breathing problems, you should have your surgery performed in a hospital so that appropriate resources are available to treat any problems that may arise.

Patient safety standards have been recently developed by several major surgery organizations and can be viewed on their Web sites (for example, the American Society of Plastic Surgeons at www.plastic surgery.org or the American College of Surgeons at www.facs.org).

Patient Education

Many surgeons provide prospective breast reduction patients with educational materials about the procedure, which may consist of illustrated pamphlets, written material developed by the surgeon's office, or a video that you view in the office or that you may be given to take home.

Informed Consent

Once you and your surgeon together have decided on a treatment plan, you will be asked to sign an informed-consent document. Before signing this document, make sure that you truly are informed: that is, your surgeon has explained and you understand the reasoning for the proposed treatment, the nature of the surgery, the risks, the benefits, and any alternatives. Some institutions require that informed-consent documents be signed within a certain time period prior to surgery, so you may not be asked to sign your consent form at the initial consultation visit. Nonetheless, you should be sure to get the information you need before you give consent.

Operative Report

Ask your surgeon to provide you with a copy of the operative report from your surgery once it becomes available. The information in the report can be very helpful to another surgeon should you need future breast surgery. Make a note to yourself to request the report again if you do not receive it within a couple of months after your surgery.

IN THE FINAL ANALYSIS . . .

Most breast reduction patients do well after surgery, but the operation is not risk free. Beyond the surgeon's good credentials and your proper medical preparation, the most important factor in determining how well you cope with surgery and treatment of any complications that may develop is the relationship between you and your surgeon. Unfortunately, doctors and patients do not have much opportunity to get to know each other prior to surgery, so you need to get a sense of the surgeon's "bedside manner" during your consultation. You should feel that you are being heard, that the surgeon understands your concerns, and that you are being taken seriously. You want a surgeon who is empathetic and not judgmental, willing to help and honest. Do *not* ask your surgeon to fabricate information in order to obtain insurance approval. You do not want his or her ethics, reputation, or credentials put at risk. Would you want a surgeon who cannot be trusted to do the right thing?

Chapter 5

Who Will Pay the Bill
Getting Insurance Coverage of Surgery

*M*any women who want to have breast reduction surgery cannot afford to proceed because they do not have insurance coverage. One of these financial scenarios probably applies to you:

SCENARIO 1 **Self pay:** You have no health insurance or you already know that you will be responsible for all expenses related to breast reduction surgery.

SCENARIO 2 **Insurance policy exclusion:** You have health insurance but breast reduction is a policy exclusion (never covered).

SCENARIO 3 **Insurance coverage per criteria:** You have health insurance with a company that will review breast reduction claims and will approve coverage if you meet specific criteria.

SCENARIO 4 **Traditional Medicare and Medicaid:** Your primary insurance is traditional (not managed care) Medicare or Medicaid.

Most health insurance policies have a list of coverage exclusions, and sometimes breast reduction surgery is on the list. More commonly, however, insurance companies perform case-by-case reviews and make determinations based on previously established criteria. It can seem a daunting task to figure out how to tackle the insurance issue, and in this chapter I will provide you with detailed advice on how to maximize the chances that your insurance company will pay for your surgery.

The most important thing that you must do, unless you are planning to pay for the surgery out of pocket, is to *find out in advance*, whenever possible, if your insurance company will cover the surgery. Have your surgeon write a letter to the insurance company detailing your relevant medical information and providing a realistic minimum estimate of the weight that he or she expects to remove from each breast. When you get an approval, make sure that you and your surgeon have the approval *in writing* so that you both know exactly what conditions, if any, have been placed on the coverage. You need to understand exactly what your financial liability will be if you do not meet those conditions after the fact. You also need to be sure that your health insurance policy will be in effect on the day of your surgery. Insurance companies have been known to refuse to pay if the surgeon does not remove the weight estimated in the preoperative letter, and they certainly will not pay if your policy is not active at the time of surgery. If you change insurance plans before your surgery date, you must start from scratch with the new company.

Even if the insurance company approves the coverage, you may still have significant out-of-pocket expenses. You may have a co-pay or a deductible, or you may be balance-billed for charges that exceed the insurance payments.

SELF PAY (SCENARIO 1)

If you do not have health insurance and do not anticipate having coverage in the near future, you will need to find out the true costs to you for the surgery. Doctors and hospitals have established charges for all procedures, but insurance companies rarely reimburse 100 percent of those charges. Both doctors and hospitals contract with insurers and agree to accept what those insurers deem to be "reasonable and customary" reimbursement. There is no universal "reasonable and customary" amount; this amount is determined unilaterally by each insurance company.

The bottom line is that if you pay the hospital 100 percent of its "retail" charge for your surgery and hospitalization, you will be their best payor by far. Therefore, you should negotiate *in advance* a fair price. Ask the surgeon about your options. Some surgeons have a standing agreement with a surgical facility for self-pay patients, in which the amount that you must pay the facility is predetermined, discounted, and conveyed to you in advance. Make sure that any quote that you receive includes *all* expected routine charges, including the preoperative area, operating room, recovery room, hospital room, drugs and intravenous fluids, anesthesia, anesthesiologist professional fees, laboratory, and pathologist professional charges. Find out what is *not* included, such as unanticipated charges for emergency care or for a hospital stay beyond what you expected (for example, if you have severe nausea and vomiting and need to stay an extra day to receive medications and intravenous fluids). You may also have to pay for extra amenities, such as television. The professional fees of the anesthesiologist and pathologist are often billed separately by those physicians and are not included in the hospital charges. If this is the case, ask your surgeon to help you get a fixed quote from these physicians. The total of the hospital charges may have to be paid in full in advance, or you may be able to set up a payment plan. Most hospitals accept credit cards, but unless you have an extremely favorable interest rate on your credit card or you are able to pay off your credit card balance right away, you can probably do better with a payment plan with the hospital than if you put the entire bill all at once on your credit card.

The forgoing advice also applies to the surgeon's fee. The national average surgeon's fee for mastopexy, a cosmetic operation similar to breast reduction, is $4,000. Self-pay breast reduction fees are likely to be in the range of $2,500 to $5,000. Find out how much care after surgery is included in the surgeon's fee. Insurance companies follow the Medicare "global period" rules, which state that routine office visits for ninety days after major surgery are covered as part of the surgery charge. However, individual surgeons may have a separate policy for self-pay patients.

Do not assume that your health insurance will kick in or that your surgeon will absorb the costs if a complication arises from what the insurance company considers cosmetic (and uncovered) surgery. Check into this ahead of time. You may be able to purchase "complications insurance" if your surgeon is enrolled in such a program.

Surgeons usually do not accept installment payments for cosmetic surgery. Some surgeons may offer an outside financing option, and you should evaluate the terms of such a plan in the same way that you would evaluate any loan offer. If you anticipate getting health insurance in the future and want to postpone having breast reduction surgery until you have coverage, do some homework ahead of time so that you do not sign up for a policy that excludes coverage of breast reduction. Also, find out if the policy includes a preexisting-conditions clause that might delay your eligibility to have breast reduction surgery covered.

INSURANCE PLANS

The rest of this chapter will discuss dealing with insurers. It may help you to understand how insurance companies handle breast reduction surgery claims if you know a little about the recent history of insurance coverage of this operation. Traditionally, insurance companies have viewed breast reduction either with skepticism as a thinly veiled cosmetic "breast lift" operation or have refused coverage because the woman was overweight. Procedures that are deemed cosmetic (primarily intended to improve someone's appearance) or that insurers feel can be treated with nonsurgical methods are often denied coverage. Insurance companies have believed and many continue to believe that breast hypertrophy (enlargement) is caused by weight gain and can be treated with weight loss. Some family doctors are not better informed and have reinforced the idea of weight loss as a treatment for large breasts. Women and their plastic surgeons know better, of course, but hard evidence that breast reduction surgery helps improve a woman's health and well-being was lacking in published reports in the medical literature until recently.

In the 1980s and 1990s, numerous reports confirming the benefits of surgery were published in the medical literature. Then two critical events occurred. In 1995, the U.S. District Court decision mentioned in Chapter Three was handed down. The judge found for the plaintiff, who had been denied insurance coverage of breast reduction surgery based on her weight, writing, ". . . the issue of whether weight loss must be attempted before breast reduction is, at least, an open question while the benefit of such a reduction to any person, has been resoundingly proven. Therefore, this court finds that the defendant's reliance on their conclusion that accepted medical practice required the plaintiff to first address her breast size by trying a more safe and conservative measure, such as weight loss, was improper."

The second milestone event was the publication in 2000 of the results of the BRAVO (Breast Reduction: Assessment of Value and Outcome) study. BRAVO was a landmark prospective study funded by the major plastic surgery professional organizations. Fourteen academic institutions participated in the BRAVO study, which included over three thousand patients. The study demonstrated unequivocally the health benefits of breast reduction surgery. Specifically, the study found that (1) women seeking breast reduction have more pain than do large-breasted women who do not seek surgery; (2) conservative (nonsurgical) therapy does not provide long-term relief of symptoms; and (3) breast reduction surgery provides substantial relief of symptoms, essentially returning women to *normal levels of functioning*. The study defined the medical (as opposed to the cosmetic) indications for surgery and found that women having two or more of the key physical symptoms (including back pain, shoulder pain, neck pain, breast pain, headaches, skin rashes, arm pain, and hand numbness) all or most of the time had the greatest health burden from their heavy breasts and were the patients most likely to have significant pain relief and improvement in physical functioning.

Internationally, breast reduction and the issue of insurance coverage have been getting attention. In Great Britain health insurance is provided by the government through the National Health Service (NHS). A study that was published in 1996 evaluated whether breast reduction surgery should be rationed by the NHS and concluded that the medical evidence supported continued coverage of the procedure by the government.

The significance of the U.S. District Court decision and the publication of the BRAVO study results is that millions of women, many of whom cannot afford to pay for major surgery out of pocket, are now more likely to be eligible for insurance coverage of breast reduction surgery and can consider surgery as a real option for treatment of their symptoms.

Insurance Policy Exclusion (Scenario 2)

Every insurance policy has an exclusions section, so look there for mention of breast reduction surgery.

I do not think that it is an overstatement to say that when it comes to health insurance benefits the number one goal of employers is to control costs. Health care is expensive and becoming more so every year. Employee health insurance is one of an employer's biggest expenses. Big companies hire benefits specialists to negotiate an employee health insurance package that will fit the budget. The benefits specialists know exactly what they are getting when they purchase a plan that specifically excludes coverage of breast reduction surgery. Smaller employers also have to worry about costs, but they may not have a dedicated benefits specialist who is as conversant with every detail of the health insurance contract.

At present, breast reduction as a policy exclusion is seen most commonly in managed-care plans (for example, HMOs). Even though this form of health insurance will probably become less common over time, other types of insurance plans may contain the same exclusion. Most health insurance plans of any type exclude coverage of cosmetic surgery, and some insurers consider breast reduction to be a cosmetic surgery, just like breast enlargement. However, physicians and patients disagree with this categorization, even though no one would deny that breast reduction does have cosmetic benefits. There are cosmetic benefits to hernia repair, but no one ever suggests that those are the primary benefits or that hernia repair should be excluded from insurance coverage. Surgical removal of an enlarged thyroid gland (goiter) also has cosmetic benefits, but I have never heard of coverage of thyroid surgery being denied for those reasons.

How can an employer justify the specific exclusion of coverage of an operation that applies only to women and that has been amply demonstrated to be *the only known effective treatment* for severe physical symptoms that impair a woman's activity level and quality of life and that prevent her from engaging in the very activities that are universally recommended by doctors and health organizations to improve her health and longevity? The ultimate irony here is that some of the very insurance companies (mainly HMOs) that on the one hand are promoting healthy lifestyles and encouraging the habit of regular exercise are on the other hand excluding coverage of an operation that allows a category of physically impaired women to participate in those healthy lifestyle activities.

Other health insurance policies may list breast reduction surgery by itself as an exclusion, separate from the cosmetic surgery category. The rationale behind this is evidently purely economic, and it does show that these companies have acknowledged that breast reduction does not fit into the cosmetic pigeonhole. In that case, what can possibly be the rationale for denying coverage across the board? I have yet to come up with a satisfactory explanation for this insurance practice. The worst aspect of this situation is that companies that exclude potentially medically necessary procedures like breast reduction surgery from coverage will not even pay for a woman to be evaluated by the appropriate specialist, no matter how severe her symptoms may be. That same woman can go, with her insurance company's approval, to an orthopedic surgeon for her shoulder pain or to a dermatologist for her skin rashes, but even if those specialists recommend that the patient have breast reduction surgery, she will not be allowed to consult with a plastic surgeon at an approved, covered visit.

If your employer provides you with health insurance benefits in which breast reduction is a policy exclusion, you and your surgeon (if you have seen one) have no recourse with the insurance company. The insurer's medical director cannot review your case. What *can* you do? Read the Denials section later in this chapter.

Insurance Coverage per Criteria (Scenario 3)

If your insurance plan covers breast reduction surgery as long as you meet the criteria, the process of obtaining coverage can be straightforward or it can be a nightmare. *You* have to be willing to make the necessary effort, and you will need your doctors (all of them) to support you. There is no guarantee that you will be successful, but this section is intended to give you as much ammunition as possible.

If your insurance policy does not specifically exclude coverage of breast reduction surgery, this implies that the company admits that breast reduction surgery *may* be medically necessary. Most companies have specific written criteria that a woman must meet. In addition, even if you and your neighbor both have health insurance through Insurance Company X, your benefit plan is very likely not the same as hers if the two of you do not have the same employer. These differences are the result of the economics of contract negotiations and have nothing to do with medical necessity. Plenty of benefits plans exclude coverage of procedures that the insurer will concede may be medically necessary.

Almost all insurance companies require prior authorization of surgeries like breast reduction. If that authorization is not obtained before the surgery is performed, the insurance company may not be obligated to pay anything, even if the surgery meets its criteria for coverage. In that situation either the patient may end up with a big bill or the surgeon and the surgical facility may be unable to collect any payment.

To obtain authorization, your surgeon should write a letter to the insurance company requesting approval of coverage of your proposed surgery. Copies of the photographs taken of you during your consultation will be included with the letter. Some surgeons require the patient to investigate her insurance coverage, and it is always helpful to read your policy or ask your benefits administrator if the surgery is covered before you ever see the surgeon. The formal request for preauthorization along with the appropriate medical information should come from the surgeon. It is also very helpful if your surgeon has a copy of your insurer's criteria for coverage for two reasons: (1) He or she can obtain from you all of the data required by the insurer; and (2) he or she may be able to speculate, based on the written criteria, whether your surgery is likely to be approved. I try to keep up to date with the current coverage criteria from the insurers that I deal with on a regular basis, although criteria can change without notice at any time from any insurer.

Unfortunately, there is a wide spectrum of insurance company criteria for coverage of breast reduction surgery. The insurance company employees who preauthorize procedures are not necessarily up to date on the most current medical evidence supporting treatment of any particular medical condition. It is the role of the insurance company's physician medical director to develop and maintain appropriate criteria to be used in claims evaluations. These physicians are not likely to be plastic surgeons! They are often trained in nonsurgical specialties and may work part time for the insurance company while continuing their own practices. Whether the medical directors are part time or full time, they may not be well versed in the current scientific literature regarding the medical indications for and the benefits of breast reduction surgery.

At the insurance company, a clerk will open the letter from the surgeon and forward it to a reviewer, often a nurse, who will either make a determination or send the request to the physician medical director. If the patient, as described by the surgeon, clearly meets the criteria for coverage, preauthorization will be given. This means that payment will be made *if* (1) the patient is still covered under the insurance plan at the time of the surgery, and (2) the extent of surgery performed is as promised, usually meaning that the weight estimated by the surgeon to be removed is in fact removed.

If a patient does not clearly meet the criteria, one of three things may happen:

1. The insurance company may approve the surgery anyway, based on the information contained in the surgeon's letter.

2. The insurer may request more information, usually about specific symptoms or prior treatment. If more information can be provided by the surgeon or the patient, a final decision will be forthcoming. If the requested information cannot be provided, a denial is likely.

3. The insurer may deny the request.

The following is a list of criteria, some combination of which is commonly used by insurers to evaluate requests for coverage:

- **Estimated weight of breast tissue to be removed.** For some companies this is the only criterion that is used to make coverage decisions. Often no other physical characteristics, such as height and body frame, are considered. The minimum qualifying weight estimate can range from 300 to 800 grams per breast (500 grams, which is slightly more than 1 pound, is common).

- **Patient's percentile on the Schnur scale,** which is based on body surface area. See page 83 for a description of the Schnur sliding scale.

- **Bra cup size.** The insurer may require that the patient currently be wearing a C cup or larger bra.

- **Body weight.** Health insurance companies commonly use life insurance tables to determine "ideal body weight" (IBW) and require a potential patient to be within a percentage of this weight. These tables compare a woman's weight to her height and body frame size (small, medium, or large). From a practical standpoint, many health insurance reviewers assume that all women have large frames, which may give you a *slight* advantage as to how heavy you can be and still be within your "ideal weight." Typically, a health insurer may require that a breast reduction candidate be within 10 percent to 30 percent of her ideal body weight. Alternatively, the insurer may base coverage decisions on body mass index (weight in kilograms divided by height in meters squared). Since over 60 percent of American women are classified as overweight or obese, an insurer who uses strict weight guidelines to assess claims will deny coverage to a large percentage of women seeking breast reduction.

- **Symptoms**

    - Back, neck, or shoulder pain that is considered to be caused by breast weight and not by other conditions. The insurer may require that the symptoms are documented to have been present for a minimum length of time, such as six months to a year, and that nonsurgical treatment, such as medication or physical therapy, has been tried and has been unsuccessful.

    - Rashes or skin breakdown under the breasts or under the bra straps that is resistant to treatment

    - Hand or arm numbness

    - Headaches

    - Painful, stooped posture (sometimes the insurer will require X-rays documenting excessive spinal curvature, or thoracic kyphosis)

    - Inability to perform one's job

- **Physical signs**

    - Large breasts

    - Shoulder grooving

- Deformity or asymmetry related to breast cancer treatment. Health insurance plans are mandated by the federal government to cover both breast reconstruction after cancer treatment and surgery on the opposite breast to obtain symmetry. This mandate supersedes policy exclusions and restrictive criteria that might otherwise prevent a woman from undergoing a breast reduction.

- **Photographs** documenting breast hypertrophy (excessive enlargement) and other signs, such as shoulder grooving, postural deformities, and skin problems

- **Documentation of failure of nonsurgical treatment.** "Conservative measures" and "medical management" usually refer to treatment recommendations such as supportive bras with wide straps, nonnarcotic pain medications, and physical therapy (including postural maneuvers and exercises). The insurer may require documentation that nonsurgical therapy has been tried for an extended period of time, such as three or six months.

- **Second opinions** may be required from the primary-care physician and/or other practitioners, such as chiropractors, rheumatologists, or orthopedic surgeons, confirming that (1) the patient's symptoms are caused by her breast size; (2) breast reduction surgery is expected to help relieve symptoms; and (3) conservative measures/medical management have been tried and have been unsuccessful.

- **Weight loss.** The insurer may require the patient to receive weight loss counseling or to document weight loss that fails to relieve symptoms. Some insurers justify the requirement for weight loss prior to surgery on the grounds that weight loss lowers the complication rate of breast reduction surgery. In fact, there is no medical evidence to support this contention.

Most insurers assign more value to certain signs and symptoms than to others, and usually multiple criteria must be fulfilled in order for the surgery to be approved. The most common criteria that I encounter are the estimate of weight to be removed, the patient's percentile on the Schnur sliding scale, and some combination of physical symptoms.

Some insurance companies specifically exclude certain complaints and symptoms as sufficient sole criteria, even if they are very distressing to the patient or despite plenty of medical evidence to indicate a relationship to breast size and weight. Examples of these exclusions that I have encountered are:

- Poor posture
- Headaches
- Difficulty finding clothes to fit
- Sagging breasts
- Distortion of the nipple/areola complex
- Skin complications unresponsive to medical management
- Inability to exercise
- Psychological or social reasons (universally rejected by insurers)

Did you notice that some of the same symptoms are listed both under accepted criteria and excluded criteria? It is possible to find an insurer who will pay for breast reduction surgery based on a single severe symptom and simultaneously identify another insurer who will not accept the same symptom, regardless of severity. This demonstrates how inconsistent the insurance industry has been in developing criteria for coverage of breast reduction surgery.

Your insurer may not respond quickly to your surgeon's letter. If no response is obtained within three weeks after the letter was sent, call your insurer to find out the status of your request. Do not wait months only to find out that the letter was lost and that you need to start over. If your surgery is approved, congratulations! As stated earlier, be sure to read the entire letter for conditions pertaining to coverage of your surgery. If coverage is denied, do not give up. You have only just begun. Read the section on denials later in this chapter.

SCHNUR SLIDING SCALE

In 1991, Dr. Paul Schnur, a plastic surgeon at the Mayo Clinic, published a scientific paper in which he described a formula that he thought would be useful for insurance companies trying to determine eligibility requirements for coverage of breast reduction surgery. He obtained information from approximately one hundred plastic surgeons about six hundred breast reduction patients, including the patients' motivations (cosmetic, medical, or both) to have surgery, their body surface areas (BSA in square meters = the square root of height in inches times weight in pounds divided by 3,131) and the weight of tissue surgically removed from their breasts. He developed a sliding scale (see Appendix A) that he believed would accurately predict which patients need surgery for medical reasons and which patients have only cosmetic reasons for wanting surgery. Although Dr. Schnur's calculations were based on actual measurements from patients who had already had surgery, the formula was proposed as a tool to be used to seek insurance approval before a woman has surgery, based on the *estimated* breast weight to be removed. Each potential candidate for breast reduction surgery falls into a particular percentile on the scale. According to the formula, a woman who falls above the 22nd percentile seeks surgery for purely medical reasons, a woman who falls below the 5th percentile seeks surgery for purely cosmetic reasons, and a woman between the 5th and 22nd percentiles has mixed reasons for wanting surgery.

Here is an example of how this formula works:

"Sara" is 5 feet 4 inches tall and weighs 180 pounds. She wears a 38DDD bra. She has a lot of back and neck pain, headaches, and shoulder grooving, and wants to have breast reduction surgery. She cannot afford to have the surgery if her insurance doesn't cover it. Her insurance company requires that her measurements put her above the 22nd percentile in order for her surgery to be covered. Her plastic surgeon estimates that he will remove about 500 grams (slightly more than 1 pound) of tissue per breast. Sara's body surface area (BSA) is 1.92 m². According to the Schnur sliding scale, Sara falls between the 5th and 22nd percentiles if her doctor removes 500 grams per breast. In that case, her insurance may deny coverage. However, if the surgeon removes an additional 50 grams per breast (the equivalent of half a stick of butter), she will exceed the 22nd percentile and her insurance company will pay.

In this scenario we will hope that the surgeon's estimate of weight to be removed was conservative and that he will be able to remove an additional 50 grams per breast safely. In some cases, however, a surgeon cannot remove any extra tissue without risking blood supply to the nipple or skin or perhaps to the detriment of the final appearance of the breast.

If you are curious about where you fall on the Schnur scale, calculate your BSA or find it on the nomogram (see Appendix A). Use the sliding scale that follows to find out how much weight your surgeon will have to remove from each breast into order to put you above the 22nd percentile. Keep in mind that 500 grams is slightly more than 1 pound. If your BSA falls between two numbers on the scale, you can split the difference in the weights that correspond with the adjacent higher and lower BSAs. However, remember that these numbers are guidelines, and some insurance companies that use the Schnur scale will give you the benefit of the weight estimate that corresponds with the lower BSA.

The value of the Schnur formula is that it gives insurance companies a tool to use to try to identify legitimate claims. In the formula the patients whose data fall below the 5th percentile have very little breast weight removed, and Dr. Schnur's survey indicated that these patients had entirely cosmetic motivations. Unfortunately, insurers do not always use the formula as it was intended and often exclude from coverage not only the patients below the 5th percentile, but also the entire group of patients between the 5th and 22nd percentiles—that is, those whose motivations include both physical and aesthetic concerns.

From a medical standpoint, the main problems with reliance on the Schnur formula are that it does not directly address the complexity of symptoms that many women face, and it takes the traditional insurance company approach of using the patient's weight and the weight of the removed tissue to make coverage determinations. Numerous recent studies have shown that women routinely underreport the severity of their symptoms and activity limitations from their breast weight, and that neither a woman's body weight nor the weight of removed tissue correlate with the benefits of breast reduction—only the severity of her symptoms predicts her result. Worst of all, the formula gives insurance companies an excuse to deny coverage to women who are deemed to have some aesthetic motivations, regardless of the severity of their physical symptoms. What is wrong with wanting your oversized, heavy breasts to look better? Does the insurance industry think that surgeons should treat the problem of heavy breasts with mastectomies and forget about trying to leave the patient with reasonably normal-looking breasts?

Despite these problems, the Schnur formula works fairly well when used as it was designed to be used. Dr. Schnur has recommended that, barring special circumstances, the women who fall above the 22nd percentile automatically receive insurance coverage of surgery and that the women who fall below the 5th percentile automatically be denied coverage. The women who fall between these points on the scale should have their claims individually reviewed for merit.

Traditional Medicare and Medicaid (Scenario 4)

Medicare is a health insurance program funded by the federal government and is available to individuals who are eligible by age or by certain disabilities. Increasing numbers of patients are enrolled in Medicare managed-care plans. Local insurance contractors administer both the traditional and the managed-care Medicare plans.

Medicaid (Title XIX of the Social Security Act) is a federal/state entitlement program that pays for medical assistance for certain individuals and families with low incomes and resources. Within broad national guidelines established by the federal government, each state establishes its own eligibility standards; determines the type, amount, duration, and scope of services; sets the rate of payment for services; and administers its own program. Medicaid policies for eligibility, services, and payment are complex and vary considerably from state to state. Medicare and Medicaid may not specifically exclude coverage of breast reduction surgery, but in my experience it has been nearly impossible to get reimbursement for the procedure when performed on patients with traditional Medicare or Medicaid insurance, even when the patient was severely symptomatic before surgery. The problem with dealing with the traditional federal or state government plans is that your surgeon probably will not be able to precertify the surgery—that is, find out ahead of time if the insurance will pay—which means that he or she may be forced to treat it as potentially medically unnecessary. In that situation you may be required to sign forms acknowledging your understanding that you may be financially liable for all of the expenses related to your surgery.

I have found that it is much easier to get approval for coverage of breast reduction for patients enrolled in managed-care Medicare or Medicaid plans. More important, these patients can seek preauthorization for surgery so that every one involved knows ahead of time if the insurance will be paying for the surgery.

DENIALS

Denial Because Breast Reduction Is a Policy Exclusion (Scenario 2)

This is the most frustrating insurance situation because women in this group, some with debilitating symptoms, are denied access to the only treatment medically proven to be effective for their problems. Most insurance companies use government-sponsored health care guidelines to develop their coverage policies, and it is quite common for insurers to provide better coverage than does the government. In this case, unfortunately, the reverse is true. Breast reduction is not a policy exclusion, nor is it considered cosmetic surgery by the government (even though from a practical perspective it is sometimes impossible to get the government to pay for it). Yet your insurance company developed a benefit package with a negotiated price tag that *specifically excludes coverage of breast reductions, and your employer bought it.* The insurer did not sneak this in, trusting no one would notice. Your employer's benefits department agreed to these terms.

Your hope in this situation is that your employer is simply unaware of the problems of heavy breasts and the medically appropriate treatment for those problems, and that your employer is willing to listen to reason and the medical evidence. Chances are that your employer thinks that a woman seeking a breast reduction either wants the surgery to improve her appearance or should lose weight if she wants her breasts to be smaller. Almost certainly your employer wants very much to reduce or at least hold steady the costs of health care for the company's employees. You may have an uphill battle. Here is your action plan:

- File an appeal with the insurance company. For a policy exclusion you will get a denial. Unless you are offered other options, file your second appeal with your state department of insurance. Your insurer will provide you with the address. This route will likely help only if your insurer is incorrect in claiming that the surgery is a policy exclusion. Some states actually mandate coverage of breast reduction surgery for women who fit criteria. If by chance you are successful in getting the department of insurance to state that breast reduction is in fact covered under your contract, you may still be told by your insurer that your case needs to go to an outside reviewer (see the section Denial [Scenario 3] on page 89).

- Find out whom in the benefits department of your company you should contact about your concerns. Present your symptoms and the medical evidence supporting breast reduction as medically necessary surgery. Include supporting letters from your family doctor, gynecologist, orthopedist, physical therapist, chiropractor, plastic surgeon—anyone who has a professional recommendation for your treatment. Put everything in writing and leave a copy with the benefits specialist.

- Pursue your employer's appeals process until it is exhausted. Be sure you have provided any information requested by your employer and have followed all of the appropriate procedures.

- If you belong to a union, ask your union representative for assistance if appropriate.

- At all times be firm but polite. **Do not make threats,** which will only halt your progress.

If you are unsuccessful with your employer you have a few options left:

- Change insurance plans at your next opportunity (usually open-enrollment periods occur annually). But be forewarned: Look before you leap. Be sure to research the likelihood of getting surgery covered under a new plan or with a new company. Naturally, you need to make certain that a new insurance plan will still give you the overall coverage that you need for other medical care.

- Get covered under someone else's policy, such as a parent or your spouse (do your homework as above).

- Change employers (again, do your homework).

- Pay for surgery on your own (read the section Self Pay [Scenario 1] at the beginning of this chapter).

- Reread Chapter 3, try to get some relief, and postpone having surgery until the financial hurdle has been overcome.

Your employer will certainly hope that you come up with an alternative that does not cost him or her more money, so it is your challenge to convince your boss that relieving your symptoms will help you become a more effective employee.

Denial Because You Do Not Meet Criteria for Coverage (Scenario 3)

Traditionally, most insurance companies have paid for breast reduction surgery for women who meet preestablished criteria. The crux of the problem for a potential patient lies in the criteria themselves.

If coverage of surgery is denied, do not give up hope. Assuming that your policy is in effect, the insurance company is denying coverage because you do not meet its criteria for coverage *based on the information provided so far.* You have the legal right to appeal this decision, and you should take advantage of the process. Many times the physician medical director for the insurance company can use some discretion in borderline cases. At other times an appeal automatically means that your request will be sent to an outside plastic surgeon for review. In any case you and/or your surgeon probably need to provide more information. Here is your action plan:

- Study the reasons for the denial, which should be provided in the denial letter. According to ERISA (Employment Retirement Income and Security Act of 1974), an insurance company is obligated to provide patients with sufficient information so that an informed appeal can be filed. The information that you need is: (1)

the specific reason for the denial; (2) the exact language in your insurance contract that applies to your request and its denial; (3) the nature of any additional information that you need to provide in order to maximize your chances of getting an eventual approval; and (4) the steps that you need to take in order to receive a review. You or your surgeon should obtain (preferably in writing) the insurer's internal guidelines that include the *exact* criteria it uses to evaluate requests for coverage of breast reduction surgery.

• Talk to your surgeon. Occasionally, the surgeon can make a phone call to the insurance company medical director and provide enough additional information to obtain an approval. If this is not an option or does not work, the two of you need to formulate a plan for your appeal.

• Based on the feedback that you have received from the insurer, you or your surgeon should provide more information. Below is a list of talking points that you and your surgeon can include in your letters. Your surgeon may have even more ammunition in his or her arsenal. At minimum the insurer should receive:

  • A letter written by you describing in detail your physical symptoms and how they have limited your activities, such as your job, schoolwork, housework, child care, or participation in sports or other recreational activities. Show the insurer how your breast size creates a disability for you. Be specific about treatments that you have tried without success. Do not make your psychological concerns the main topic of your letter. (These issues are important to you, but they will carry little if any weight with the insurer, and overemphasis on them may lessen the impact of your description of your physical problems.)

  • Supporting letters from any physician or therapist that you have seen for your symptoms. These letters should be detailed and should contain information on your symptoms and physical findings, the length of time you have complained of your symptoms, all treatments prescribed, the results of treatment, and any recommendations (which presumably will include breast reduction).

In some cases it may be appropriate to include supporting letters from your employer, military commander, or any other person whose duty it is to evaluate your job performance and your ability to perform any and all aspects of your job.

If your surgeon plans to write an appeal letter, he or she should include the above-mentioned supporting documents. Otherwise you can submit them yourself along with your appeal.

- You or your representative should file the actual appeal with the insurer. You can authorize anyone do this for you, and your surgeon may be in a good position to do so if he or she has more information to send. As stated above, your denial letter from the insurance company should have included instructions on how to file an appeal. If it did not, check your policy handbook or call the insurance company directly. Find out the proper address to which you should send your appeal. A typical appeals process works like this:

  1. You register your appeal by sending a letter to the insurance company stating why you disagree with its decision to deny coverage of surgery and why you think it should change its decision.

  2. At most insurance companies a physician will perform the first, *internal* review of an appeal for denial of coverage. You should receive a response in writing within a reasonable time period, such as four to six weeks.

  3. If you receive a second denial you can request an *external* review by an outside organization, i.e., one not affiliated with your insurance company. You usually have to request this review within a certain time frame, such as within sixty days. Most states provide patients with the right to an external review, even if the insurance plan does not include this option.

  4. In some states external review decisions are binding, while in other states they are advisory. The outside reviewer will either reverse your insurer's decision, in which case your surgery may be covered, or will agree with your insurer, in which case you will probably have to find another source of payment. You can look up your state's regulations on this issue at www.nahu.org/government/charts.htm.

- Take full advantage of the appeals process. This is your right, and patients who are committed to the process are often successful in achieving their goals. You may be entitled to attend a hearing at some level of the appeals process, and you should do so. Your surgeon does not need to attend the hearing unless he or she can make a contribution in person that could not be made in writing.

- If at the end of the appeals process you still have not received an approval of coverage, you can pursue the options listed earlier for denials because of a policy exclusion. Alternatively, you can pursue legal avenues. The woman in Michigan who took her case to the U.S. District Court in 1996 won her case. By then she had already taken out a loan and undergone surgery, but she was asking for reimbursement from the insurer.

Medicare and Medicaid Denials (Scenario 4)

In my experience patients with traditional Medicare insurance have not been able to obtain predetermination reviews of their requests for payment of breast reduction surgery. This means that unless the patient signs a waiver before surgery stating that she knows Medicare may not cover her surgery and that she accepts financial responsibility, the surgeon and the facility risk not being able to collect anything. Many surgeons and hospitals do not want to take that risk, and many Medicare patients also do not want to risk being responsible for the thousands of dollars that breast reduction surgery is likely to cost. Medicare does have an appeals process that can be used after surgery if payment is denied, but this process can be drawn out and difficult.

Patients who are enrolled in Medicare managed-care plans and who are denied coverage of breast reduction surgery can appeal to the Center for Health Dispute Resolution (CHDR), which contracts with The Centers for Medicare and Medicaid Services (CMS, formerly HCFA) to complete reconsideration and review of determination decisions made by private insurers regarding their Medicare enrollees. Since breast reduction is considered medically necessary in cases that meet criteria, a reversal of an HMO's denial by the CHDR is final and binding, and means that the HMO must pay for the surgery.

Medicaid rules vary from state to state and, as with Medicare, it is difficult to get breast reduction surgery paid for by the government if a woman is covered by a traditional plan. Medicaid HMOs (like Medicare HMOs) may be more likely to pay and usually will do predeterminations, so that if coverage is denied you can find that out before surgery is performed. Talk to your surgeon about how to proceed if you get a Medicaid HMO denial. In most cases you will follow the same procedures that you would for a denial based on failure to meet criteria (Scenario 3).

Appeal Letter Talking Points

When you write your appeal letter, be sure to discuss your physical symptoms and limitations. You or your surgeon or both of you should point out the critical issues regarding breast hypertrophy, such as:

- There is considerable medical evidence that breast reduction surgery helps women with physical symptoms related to their breast size. The results of surgery are best predicted by the severity of the symptoms and not by the patient's preoperative bra cup size, body weight, or the weight of the tissue removed.

- There is no medical evidence that conservative measures taken to relieve the symptoms of heavy breasts offer any long-term benefit. These measures include weight loss, which has never been shown to decrease breast size reliably or to alleviate the symptoms of large breasts.

- The National Institutes of Health and most insurance companies properly stress exercise as a key component of a healthy lifestyle, yet studies have repeatedly shown that many breast reduction candidates cannot exercise effectively or even perform routine daily tasks because of symptoms related to their breast size. If you get a denial, you might want to research your insurer's position on exercise so that you can point out how patients are getting contradictory messages. (The patient publications of one of our local insurance companies demonstrate the irony of its emphasis on exercise. This particular company has an extensive series of articles on its Web site that promote exercise as a way to reduce the risk of many serious medical problems, reduce stress, and increase endurance. The Web site lists low-intensity activities that are less beneficial but still helpful, such as walking, gardening, and housework, and states that the risks of a lifestyle without exercise far outweigh the risks of exercise. Yet this same company has a policy exclusion of coverage of breast reduction, thus denying their women subscribers who cannot walk for any length of time *or* garden *or* do housework because of their breast weight the only medical treatment known to provide permanent relief of their symptoms.) Several studies of women who have had breast reduction surgery have shown dramatic increases in activity levels. One study showed that the percentage of these women who could not participate in sports increased from 5 percent before surgery to 90 percent after surgery.

- Breast reduction surgery (as opposed to mastopexy or breast lift) is not cosmetic surgery, even though it may have cosmetic benefits. Its purpose is to relieve the symptoms caused by heavy breasts. The American Medical Association adopted the following definitions of cosmetic and reconstructive surgery in 1989: Cosmetic surgery is performed to reshape normal structures of the body in order to improve the patient's appearance and self-esteem. Reconstructive surgery is performed on abnormal structures of the body, caused by congenital defects, developmental abnormalities, trauma, infection, tumors, or disease. It is generally performed to improve function, but may also be done to approximate a normal appearance.

The appeal letter should seek to educate the insurance company about the current medical literature supporting the medical benefits of breast reduction surgery. A list of some of the most recent articles on the subject can be found in the bibliography at the end of this book.

Chapter 6
Getting Ready
Preparing for Surgery

*Y*ou have made your decision to have surgery, and now it is time for you to do everything that you can to help ensure that you have a smooth surgical experience and a swift recovery. I know from years of experience that women who prepare physically, logistically, and psychologically for breast reduction surgery give themselves a big head start in the recovery process.

MONTHS AND WEEKS BEFORE SURGERY

Physical Preparation

TAKE CHARGE OF YOUR BODY

Quit Smoking

Smoking puts carbon monoxide and nicotine (among other chemicals) into your body, and there is plenty of scientific evidence that smoking impairs healing by reducing blood flow and oxygen to tissues. In breast reduction surgery, the nipple is at particular risk because part of its blood supply is surgically disrupted. Smoking further increases the risk that the nipple won't heal well or, in the worst situation, won't survive. The detrimental effects of smoking take months to reverse themselves, so even if you are just thinking about having surgery, *quit now*. Talk to your family doctor if you need help. You should wean yourself off all nicotine products before surgery.

Stop Using Recreational Drugs

If you use street drugs, be sure to tell your surgeon, for the same reasons that you should report your alcohol consumption habits (see page 100). Do not use any stimulating or intoxicating substances or drugs for at least one week before surgery.

Avoid Tanning

Tanning damages your skin and impairs healing. Take special precautions to avoid tanning and sunburns to your chest skin for at least one month before surgery.

Nutrition and Diets

Good nutrition prior to surgery is essential. Eat a well-balanced diet. If you want to lose weight before surgery, by all means go for it. However, you do not want to go on a stringent or "crash" diet or start taking diet pills. If you want to lose significant amounts of weight first, postpone the surgery until you are near your weight goal and are eating a well-balanced maintenance diet. Definitely avoid ephedra, phenylpropanolamine (PPA), fenfluramine, dexfenfluramine, and fen-phen, since all of these drugs have been shown to have dangerous side effects, especially during anesthesia.

Rest

Make sure that you are getting enough sleep. You do not want to add the stress of surgery to a body that is already exhausted.

Exercise

Many large-breasted women find it difficult to exercise, but if walking is all that you can do, *do it* and do it every day. If you build up strength in your leg muscles, you will be much less tired and will recover faster after surgery.

WORK WITH YOUR DOCTORS

Many of my breast reduction patients have medical problems, but nonetheless they do very well with surgery. After the surgeon has reviewed your medical history, he or she will make recommendations that will prepare you for the operation. You may need basic testing, which may include a blood test for hemoglobin level and, depending on your age and medical conditions, a pregnancy test, mammogram, chest X-ray, EKG, and additional blood work.

Most breast reduction patients do not require blood transfusion. In a rare situation, a surgeon may anticipate a greater than usual blood loss, and the patient may be asked either to donate a unit of her own blood in advance of surgery or to undergo blood testing (type and crossmatch) in anticipation of possible blood transfusion. If you are faced with this situation, you may wish to ask family members to donate blood intended for your use. Ask your surgeon, local Red Cross, or blood bank how to arrange this type of directed donation. Your family member's blood will be fully tested and can be released for use by another patient if you do not need it.

If your insurance is covering your surgery, it should also cover all of your testing, as long as the testing is medically necessary and appropriate. Some younger patients may have trouble getting mammograms covered. Check with your insurance company if you are not sure.

If you have any of the medical conditions or risk factors listed in Chapter 4, you and/or your surgeon should make arrangements to:

Stop Certain Medications

Many medications, including vitamins and over-the-counter drugs, can interfere with normal blood clotting. Nutritional supplements and herbals can interfere with many important body functions, including blood clotting. Table 6–1 lists common prescription and nonprescription medications that ideally should be discontinued at least two weeks prior to surgery. Table 6–2 lists some of the popular herbals that should be discontinued at least one week before surgery. If you take a medication that is not on this list, check the package insert or with your family doctor or pharmacist to find out if the drug can cause bleeding. In general, classes of drugs that should be stopped are **blood thinners, aspirin, Vitamin E, and nonsteroidal anti-inflammatory drugs (NSAIDs).** Some prescription drugs on the list may cause problems if they are stopped abruptly. Ask your surgeon if they need to be stopped at all, and then ask the prescribing physician how to do so safely. Products containing acetaminophen (for example, Tylenol) do not need to be discontinued.

Table 6–1 **Drugs That Can Cause Bleeding**

Generic or chemical names are in lower case. Brand names are in upper case. Both prescription and nonprescription drugs are listed. Most, but not all, of these drugs are blood thinners or anti-inflammatories. This is not a complete list, and new drugs come on the market frequently. During the writing of this book, one prescription anti-inflammatory (Vioxx) was taken off the market and several other prescription and nonprescription anti-inflammatories were receiving increased scrutiny by the FDA in relation to possible increased risk of heart attack.

Adalat	Clinoril	Ginseng	Nuprin	sulindac
Advil	clopidogrel	ibuprofen	Orudis	Ticlid
Aggrenox	Congespirin	Indocin	Oruvail	ticlopidine
Agrylin	Coumadin	indomethacin	Paroxetine	Tolectin
Aleve	coumarin	Jantoven	Paxil	Toradol
Alka-Seltzer	diclofenac	Lodine	pentoxifylline	Trental
Anacin	diflunisal	meloxicam	Percodan	Trilisate
Anaprox	dipyridamole	Midol	Persantine	valdecoxib
Arthrotec	Dolobid	Mobic	piroxicam	Vanquish
aspirin	Ecotrin	Motrin	Plavix	venlafaxine
Bextra	Empirin	nabumetone	Pletal	Vicoprofen
Bufferin	Excedrin	Naprelan	Ponstel	Vioxx
Cataflam	Feldene	Naprosyn	Pravigard	Vitamin E
Celebrex	Fiorinal	naproxen	Procardia	Voltaren
celecoxib	Garlic	nifedipine	Relafen	warfarin
cilostazol	Ginkgo biloba	Norgesic	rofecoxib	

Table 6–2 **Herbals**

These herbals can cause serious complications with general anesthesia and surgery and should be stopped at least one week before surgery.

Aloe vera	Ginseng
Echinacea	Kava
Ephedra	St.-John's-wort
Garlic	Valerian
Ginkgo	

Prescribe Steroids

If you have taken steroid pills (e.g., Prednisone) for any reason within the past year, you may need to receive replacement steroid medication before and after your surgery. Prolonged steroid use causes suppression of normal steroid production by your adrenal glands. Natural steroids are a critical component of the body's response to stress, and if your adrenal glands are not producing enough of them, you may have trouble with blood pressure or other problems during and after surgery. One or more doses of intravenous steroid medication can help prevent those problems.

Adjust the Surgery Date Due to Prior Accutane Use

Accutane is a powerful Vitamin A derivative that is prescribed for the treatment of severe acne. Accutane impairs skin-wound healing, and its effects linger for months. If you have been using Accutane within the past year, be sure to let your surgeon know. I recommend that patients be completely off Accutane for three to six months before having surgery of any kind.

Avoid Drugs Causing Allergic Reactions

Your surgeon will make the necessary adjustments if you are allergic to any of the medications that he or she routinely prescribes. Be sure to identify any oral pain medications or antibiotics to which you are allergic so that appropriate prescriptions will be given to you after surgery.

Schedule a Latex-Free Environment

Many surgery facilities are switching to latex-free products, but you need to inform your surgeon if you have or suspect that you have a latex (natural rubber) allergy. Latex allergy reactions include skin rashes; hives; nasal, eye, or sinus symptoms; asthma; and (rarely) shock. The operating room staff will substitute latex-free products as required. Some facilities request that a patient with a latex allergy be the first case of the day in the assigned operating room.

Avoid Other Allergenic Substances

Many items other than latex that are used in hospitals can cause problems for susceptible individuals, such as adhesive monitor patches and surgical wash solutions. Be sure to notify your surgeon if you have a particular sensitivity.

Take into Account Your Alcohol Use

If you regularly drink large amounts of alcohol, you will handle anesthetic and pain control drugs differently than do other patients. You will also be at increased risk for bleeding problems. Make your physician aware of your drinking history. All patients should avoid alcoholic beverages for twenty-four to forty-eight hours before surgery.

Document the Status of Heart Problems

Your surgeon and the anesthesiologist may want a cardiologist to document whether you have heart problems that might increase your risks with general anesthesia. If you have known heart problems, you may be asked to obtain a current assessment. Mitral valve prolapse (MVP) is a heart valve condition that is frequently diagnosed in younger patients. If you have MVP, particularly if you have symptoms, you may receive intravenous antibiotics prior to and during surgery.

Treat High Blood Pressure

Patients with uncontrolled hypertension need to get their blood pressure into normal range before undergoing elective surgery. Good control of your blood pressure is critical during breast reduction surgery in order to minimize blood loss and other complications. The anesthesiologist may want you to take your usual blood pressure medication on the morning of surgery with a sip of water. Find out in advance what you should do.

Eliminate or Minimize Breathing Problems

Breathing problems need to be aggressively evaluated and treated before you can undergo general anesthesia for elective surgery. As with heart problems, you may need to see a specialist for testing and treatment before surgery can be scheduled. If you have asthma that is under good control, the anesthesiologist can give you breathing treatments while you are asleep that will help prevent wheezing and coughing. These treatments can be continued as needed while you are in the hospital.

Wait for Respiratory Infections to Clear Before Having Surgery

If you develop a cold, sinus infection, cough, or other respiratory symptoms prior to surgery, check with the surgeon's office. Your surgery will be cancelled if you arrive at the hospital with significant respiratory symptoms.

Evaluate Prior Personal or Family Problems with Anesthesia

You may not meet the anesthesiologist until the day of surgery, so tell the surgeon in advance of any problems that you or family members have had with general or local anesthesia, in case advance preparation is warranted.

Order Preventative Measures for Blood Clots

If you or family members have a history of blood clots in the legs or abdomen (deep venous thrombosis, or DVT), your risk is increased for having a similar problem during any surgery. Tell your plastic surgeon if any family members have died suddenly right after surgery or childbirth. (This is a common presentation of pulmonary embolism, or a blood clot that lodges in an artery to the lungs.) Other factors that increase the risk of blood clots include extreme obesity; recent injury; any disorder of the heart, lungs, or central nervous system; a history of cancer, recurrent severe infection or genetic problems that affect blood clotting; current or recent use of oral contraceptives; and ongoing hormone-replacement therapy. Safety measures to prevent blood clots will be instituted according to your individual degree of risk. A woman with moderate to high risk may wear special inflatable cuffs on her calves to keep the blood in her veins moving during and immediately after surgery, and she may be instructed to wear elastic stockings for a short period after surgery. In rare cases blood-thinning medications or more complex preventative measures may be recommended, although many surgeons will be reluctant to perform breast reduction surgery on a patient who requires blood thinners.

Optimize Diabetes Control

If you have diabetes, your blood sugar will be checked before and after surgery. If you normally take insulin, your regular morning dose may be reduced for the morning of surgery, and adjustments will be made for future doses until you resume your regular eating pattern. The physician who treats your diabetes should be consulted ahead of time to handle these issues. *Be sure to find out in advance how much insulin you should take on the morning of surgery.*

Treat Severe Anemia

There can be moderate blood loss during a breast reduction, and your hemoglobin level may drop slightly after surgery. If your hemoglobin is already low, your blood will be able to carry less oxygen to the surgery site for healing. You should undergo treatment of any significant anemia before surgery. Some surgeons routinely prescribe iron pills for their breast reduction patients to help restore blood oxygen-carrying capacity.

Stop Blood-Thinner Medications and Evaluate Bleeding Problems

If you or anyone in your family has ever had a bleeding problem, your surgeon will need more information before determining if you should undergo breast reduction surgery. If you take a blood thinner, such as Coumadin, you will most likely have to stop this medication for several days before and after surgery. You or the surgeon's office staff should contact the doctor who orders your medication to determine if it is safe for you to stop it. You also should stop taking any other medicine that could interfere with blood clotting (Table 6–2).

Protect Implanted Devices or Prostheses with Antibiotics

If you have an implanted device, you will most likely be given intravenous antibiotics to minimize the risk of infection around internal foreign bodies, such as artificial joints, pacemakers, or artificial heart valves.

Postpone Surgery for Recent Pregnancy or Breastfeeding

You should not plan breast reduction surgery if you are pregnant or are trying to get pregnant, unless it is an emergency (see Chapter 11). Elective surgery during pregnancy poses unnecessary risks to the baby and to the patient. If you become pregnant during the planning phase of your breast reduction, surgery should be postponed. I do not perform breast reduction surgery on a recently pregnant or lactating woman until at least six months have passed since delivery *and* she has *completely* stopped nursing. The reason is that breasts maintain a tremendously increased blood supply during pregnancy and lactation, and even occasional nursing maintains this blood supply. Breast surgery during this time can be accompanied by an undesirable level of blood loss. Once nursing stops, the breast blood supply starts to diminish, and after six months it returns to near its prepregnancy condition. Some women may still notice occasional milk leakage from their nipples for more than a year, but this is not a cause for concern.

Consider History of Breast Cancer and Its Treatment

If breast reduction surgery is to be performed on a breast cancer patient, the surgeon may need to adapt the reduction operation to take into account how the cancer was treated (see Chapter 11).

Consider Prior Breast Surgery

Prior surgery on your breasts may have disrupted a portion of their blood supply and may put your nipples at increased risk. Your surgeon may need more information about the previous surgery, in particular the operative report, in order to plan a safe operation.

Eliminate Breast and Skin Infections

Infections of the breast itself are uncommon and must be treated aggressively and completely before surgery can be performed. Rashes and skin infections around and under the breast are common, but also need to be treated aggressively to minimize the chances of a surgical infection. The strategy to fight breast-crease infections is to control moisture with powder (baby powder, cornstarch, or medicated powders) and to treat bacterial or fungal infections with topical medications. Occasionally, oral antibiotics are prescribed.

Evaluate and Stabilize Chronic Infectious Conditions

The surgeon may request that a patient with a chronic infectious viral disease have a current examination and appropriate testing by the treating physician to assess activity of the disease. Hospital personnel may need to employ special procedures during surgery, such as double-gloving, in order to minimize the risks of disease transmission.

Prevent Urination or Bladder Problems

If you have trouble emptying your bladder, you are likely to experience urinary retention after general anesthesia. This problem can be treated with a bladder catheter if necessary. Tell your surgeon if you are prone to urinary tract infections so that you can be prescribed the appropriate antibiotics if needed.

Assess Eating Disorders

A patient with an eating disorder may or may not be a candidate for breast reduction surgery. This subject is discussed in Chapter 11.

Discuss Psychological Problems or Psychiatric Treatment

Like all surgery, breast reduction can create psychological stress. Be sure to tell your surgeon about any past and current psychological problems that you may have.

Discuss Religious/Traditional/Ethnic/Cultural Issues

Some patients have nonmedical concerns that may influence the surgeon's decision making. Most of the time, satisfactory alternatives to the usual routine can be implemented or may already be in place. For example, my hospital has a bloodless care program that was specifically designed to meet the needs of Jehovah's Witnesses. Potential issues in this broad category should be discussed with your surgeon and addressed in advance as needed.

It should go without saying that if you have any significant medical issues that are not mentioned in this chapter, you need to discuss them with your surgeon.

Logistical Preparation

Women can't just take time off work and be ready for surgery. We are usually the chief cooks and bottle washers, so to speak, so we have to arrange for child care, figure out who will do the laundry and the housework, and find a driver. We also have to find someone who can take care of *us* while we're out of commission. If you deal with these issues before surgery, you will have made the difference between an easy and an extremely stressful recovery. Find out how much your spouse can be counted on to do. Prevail on your family and friends to volunteer their services. Temporary live-in help is great, especially if you have small children.

TIME OFF WORK

I recommend that breast reduction patients plan to take two weeks off work for a desk job, four weeks for a job that requires moderate to heavy lifting, and six weeks for a job that is very strenuous. It may help you to ease back into your work routine by planning to return in the middle of your work week. Some patients may be able to return to work sooner than expected, and patients who experience delays in healing or other complications may have to stay off work longer. Obtain any forms that your employer requires in order to document your request for medical leave so that you can receive any benefits to which you are entitled. Fill out your portion of the forms before you give them to the surgeon's office staff. Find out if you will be permitted to return to work if you have restrictions or limitations. Some employers are able to modify jobs so that temporarily disabled employees can return to work before they are able to resume their regular job duties.

DRIVING

Arrange for someone to drive you home after surgery. I recommend that patients should not drive for one week after surgery and limit driving to short trips during the second week.

HOUSEWORK AND MEAL PREPARATION

It doesn't do you any good to stay off work if you use your recovery time to clean out the closets and wash all the rugs. Do not plan to do anything more strenuous than making yourself a sandwich during the first two weeks after surgery. Do not do laundry or push the sweeper. Let someone else do the cooking or get take-out food. *Read this paragraph again on day seven after surgery!* The first week does not present a problem because patients are sore and do not feel like doing much. Emotional and physical symptoms, including weepiness, depression, and overtiredness, tend to arise the second week, when patients are starting to feel better physically and try to do too much. Remember: Surgery is just as stressful as any major injury, and you need to give your body enough time and rest to get a good start on the healing process. I always tell my patients that if they lie low for two full weeks, their total recovery period will be much shorter than if they do too much too soon.

CHILDREN

The typical breast reduction patient is not hospitalized for more than twenty-four hours, but this may be the first time that she has spent the night away from her children. Young children, especially those younger than kindergarten age, need to be reassured about what is happening, and you should arrange for plenty of extra help during your recovery. Tell children in advance something to the effect that "Mommy is going to the hospital for a short time, she will be back very soon, and she will be fine but will not be able to pick you up or give big hugs for a little while until her 'boo-boo' gets better." *You* know that you will need to protect your incisions and should not do any significant lifting for several weeks, but your toddler will not understand why he cannot sit on Mommy's lap or why you cannot lift him out of his crib. If you take the time to explain your limitations to your children, they will be less likely to feel that they are being rejected or punished for some misbehavior. Do not give a young child any specific details. Children in this age group commonly have mutilation anxieties, and they should not be exposed to surgical wounds or dressing changes.

WOUND CARE

You may find it helpful to use a shower chair for a week or so, especially if taking narcotics makes you feel lightheaded. You can probably change your own dressings, but it is easier if you have help, especially if you have drainage tubes or develop any wound complications. Find out in advance if your spouse will be able to provide this assistance (not all men can deal with nursing duties). If he cannot help, enlist the aid of a family member or friend—it doesn't have to be someone with medical training. Your surgeon will give you specific wound-care instructions. I allow my patients to shower the day after surgery. We use sterile surgical gauze for dressings in the hospital, but for home care I recommend disposable menstrual and nursing pads that are cheap, readily available, highly absorbent, and can be tucked into your bra. Pads with adhesive strips are best for staying in place. You may want to stock up on these supplies before surgery (this avoids your husband having to buy them, which most men hate to do).

Psychological Preparation

If you are physically prepared for surgery and have dealt with all of the logistical issues, you are ahead of the game. Along the way you should assess your psychological preparedness. You do not want to get bogged down with other details only to discover at the last minute that you have a lot of unanswered questions. Here are a few questions you should ask yourself:

AM I FULLY INFORMED?

You got information from your surgeon, and there is a lot of information in this book. You may feel overwhelmed or that you really don't need all this detail. Or perhaps you have some burning questions that have not been addressed. Do not hesitate to call the surgeon's office with your questions. If you have a lot of questions or just want to listen to the surgeon explain the procedure again, ask to make an appointment for a second consultation. (Find out if there is a charge for the second visit so that there will be no misunderstanding.)

IS MY SIGNIFICANT OTHER ON BOARD?

A man sometimes has a hard time with the idea that the woman in his life wants smaller breasts (see Chapter 11). Over the years I have met many wonderful and supportive husbands of breast reduction patients, and they deserve much of the credit for their wives' swift recovery after surgery. The reality is that not all men respond in such a positive way. Talk to your partner about your surgery. Explain to him the problems that you are having and how they are affecting your life. Show him the grooves in your shoulders. If you want him to accompany you to your consultation with the surgeon, don't wait for him to volunteer: Ask him to go with you. Encourage him to tell you honestly how he feels about your having the surgery. Make sure that he has an opportunity to express those feelings to the surgeon, if he wishes, and to ask questions. During the planning phase prior to surgery, make a list of all the chores, child care, and transportation issues that have to be addressed, and find out exactly how much he is willing and able to do. Ask him if he is willing to help you with wound care and dressing changes. Make sure that *you* understand what your limitations will be after surgery, so that you will know how much he can be counted on to do and how much extra help you will need. Finally, remember that this is *your* decision to make. No one, not even your doctors, truly knows what it is like to live with the weight of your breasts. Your partner should appreciate your including him in the decision-making process, but he should respect your right to make the final decision on your own.

Some women have other family members who have strong objections to the idea of their having breast reduction surgery. If you have a close relative (for example, your father or mother) who does not support you and whose input is important to you, ask him or her to come to the first or second consultation visit with you. Sometimes just getting more information can help that family member understand and support you. Inform the surgeon of any family-support issues that may compromise your ability to do well after surgery.

WHAT DO I WANT OTHERS TO KNOW?

Some women want to keep their surgery a complete secret. Others welcome the support they receive from family, friends, and/or co-workers. The choice is yours. Your physicians and your employer are obligated by law to protect your privacy and may release your medical information without your permission only under very limited conditions (mainly in order to process your insurance claim). Sharing your story encourages other women with the same problem to seek help. If you prefer not to reveal that you had breast reduction surgery, say nothing. People may notice that you look different, but chances are they won't be able to pinpoint exactly why. If they comment, you can truthfully reply that you have lost weight and then change the subject.

WHAT AM I AFRAID OF?

I see each of my breast reduction patients a week or two before surgery to give her an opportunity to ask questions or to bring in her partner or parent, if we haven't met before. Usually the patient tells me she is nervous and I smile and answer, "That's normal!" And it is. Apprehension is a completely natural emotion prior to surgery and general anesthesia. Undoubtedly, you are concerned about how your breasts will look after surgery. Some surgeons show pictures of other patients' results, although you must keep in mind that all women are different and no specific shape, size, or scar quality can be guaranteed. Here are a few things to remember that may help ease your anxiety:

- Modern general anesthesia is very safe.
- Breast surgery is not as painful as childbirth or major organ surgery, and you will get a prescription for pain medication.
- You do not need to look at your breasts or at your incisions until you are ready. If this is a big concern, ask a friend to help you with dressing changes.
- The vast majority of women are very happy with the results of their breast reduction surgery and would choose it again or recommend it to others.

Financial Preparation

If you are paying for the surgery yourself, be sure that you understand and meet the payment schedule. Most surgeons will cancel a surgery date if an advance payment is delinquent. If you are counting on your insurance company to pay the bill, now is the time to make sure that (1) the insurance company has approved coverage of your surgery; (2) you (and/or your surgeon) have this approval *in writing;* and (3) there is a clear understanding by all parties of any limiting conditions of the approval. For example, your insurer may require that you have your surgery performed as an outpatient, that you get a second opinion, or that a minimum weight be removed (see Chapter 5).

THE WEEK BEFORE SURGERY

Now that your surgery date is near, it is time to review your final "to do" list. Paying attention to these last-minute details can help smooth your surgery and recovery experience:

Be sure that your surgeon has your *current* medical history.

It may be weeks since you last saw your surgeon. Be sure to notify the surgeon's office of *any* recent changes in your medical condition, including but not limited to new diagnoses, new medications, new allergies (especially to medications), and infections.

Treat rashes.

If you have rashes under your breasts, hopefully you have been treating them before now. Tell your surgeon if the rashes persist. You may need a prescription medication.

Take prescribed medications.

If your surgeon has given you prescriptions for medications to be taken after surgery, get them filled now.

Collect supplies.

- **Antibacterial soap**

- **Dressings:** Stock up on the wound care supplies recommended by your surgeon.

- **Sports bras:** You will most likely get bras at the time of surgery, but it is helpful to have a sports bra (or two) available that you know is comfortable. Choose one that fastens in the front. Buy one that fits you *now*, since you will have dressings that take up the extra space.

- **Old clothes:** Set aside some loose shirts that do not have to go over your head and that can be discarded if they get bloodstains on them.

- **Frozen peas and small plastic freezer bags:** Frozen peas make good ice packs. Buy a big bag of frozen peas and a box of one-quart recloseable plastic bags. The freezer bags are sturdier and work best. Fill half a dozen of the small bags about half full with peas and put them back in the freezer.

- **Shower chair:** You can pick one up at a medical supply rental company or borrow one, or (if you have room) you can use a plastic lawn chair or stool.

Review your instructions.

My patients get four pages of instructions that cover what to do before surgery, what to expect on the day of surgery, and what to do after surgery. Each patient receives this packet in advance so that most of her questions are answered before she gets to the hospital. If your surgeon gives you specific instructions, go over them again and get answers to any questions that you may still have.

Start washing.

I recommend that patients wash with an antibacterial soap starting two days before surgery.

Pack a bag.

- Pack a small overnight bag. Include or plan to wear to the hospital comfortable clothes that do not go on over your head. Do not bring a nightgown or pajamas, which could get ruined from bloody drainage. You will be given a patient gown that makes the examination of your surgery site easier.

- In your bag include your regular prescription medications in their labeled pharmacy bottles.

- You may want to take your own pillow with an old pillowcase (or you can get a pillowcase from the hospital).

- Pack light. Unless the surgery facility has secure storage space, everything you bring with you will have to stay with a companion until your room is ready after surgery.

TWENTY-FOUR HOURS BEFORE SURGERY
Identify your whereabouts.

Unfortunately, last-minute schedule changes do happen, so make sure that your surgeon is able to contact you if necessary. Also, confirm that your surgeon's office has the name and correct telephone number where you can be reached after surgery. Your cell phone number is not enough.

Nothing to eat or drink after midnight tonight.

Avoid alcohol for at least twenty-four hours before surgery.

Alcohol promotes bleeding and can interfere with anesthetic drugs.

Arrange for someone to drive you home at the time of your discharge from hospital or surgery facility.

THE MORNING OF SURGERY

Today is the day! Just a few last-minute reminders:

- ☐ Be sure not to eat or drink *anything*.
- ☐ Take only those medications that you were *specifically instructed to take on the morning of surgery*. Diabetics generally take half their usual insulin dose, and your particular instructions should have been clarified before now. If you were specifically told to take any medication by mouth this morning, take it with a small sip of water.
- ☐ Leave all valuables, jewelry, money, and contact lenses at home!
- ☐ Wear your glasses and bring a case for storage.
- ☐ If you have dentures, wear them.
- ☐ Do not wear makeup.
- ☐ Do not bring small children to the hospital with you.
- ☐ Be sure to arrive at the facility on time. This may be up to two hours before the actual surgery start time. Patients for elective surgery who arrive late run the risk of having their surgery canceled.

KEYS TO A SUCCESSFUL OUTCOME

If you have read this far and feel overwhelmed by the amount of information in this chapter, you might be wondering what are truly the most important things that you can do to maximize your chances of having a successful surgical outcome. I think that it is possible to boil down all of this information into a few key concepts:

- Become a well-informed patient.

- Pick a qualified, experienced surgeon.

- Let the surgeon help you decide if you are a suitable candidate for surgery.

- Understand the potential benefits and limits of surgery.

  - Have realistic expectations: Do not expect perfection.

  - Know that your results may not be exactly as you imagined.

- Know the risks of surgery.

- Take charge of your body—control risk factors that you can control.

- Be prepared for some pain, discomfort, and inconvenience.

- Arrange to have enough help after surgery.

- Avoid undergoing surgery during a stressful period in your life.

- Know and be prepared to fulfill your financial obligations.

- Commit to following your surgeon's instructions.

Read the next chapter to find out what actually happens at the surgery facility, from the time you arrive until your surgery is completed.

Chapter 7

In the Operating Room
What Happens on
the Day of Surgery

$\mathcal{I}$f you ask ten plastic surgeons how they do a breast reduction operation, you'll probably get ten different answers. Breast reduction surgery has been performed for 150 years, and dozens of techniques have been described and refined. These techniques get passed down to each new generation of plastic surgeons–in–training (residents or fellows), who in turn refine them further through experience. Your surgeon will choose an operation with which he or she is comfortable and that is appropriate for you.

BEFORE YOUR ANESTHESIA

When you arrive at the surgery facility, you will register and complete necessary paperwork. Your companions will not be able to accompany you to surgery or to the recovery area, but will have an opportunity to talk to the surgeon when your operation is finished. Family members and other companions who plan to wait should sign in at the waiting room desk and may be offered a pager. If none of them plan to stay, be sure to tell the facility staff who you wish them to contact when the surgery is completed.

After registration you will be escorted to the preoperative (or holding) area and will change into a patient gown. Nurses and the doctor who will be giving your anesthesia will evaluate you to confirm that you are properly prepared for surgery. Your surgeon will ask you to stand or sit upright so that he or she can measure and mark where your breast incisions will be made and where the new nipple positions will be. You will have an intravenous (IV) catheter inserted into a hand or arm vein so that you can receive fluids during surgery. You will have patches placed on your skin so that your heart can be monitored and a clip placed on your finger to measure the oxygen in your blood. You may receive a sedative medication in your IV to help relax you prior to going to the operating room. If this is offered, ask to use the bathroom first. Once you get to the operating room, your monitor patches and clips will be adjusted, and you will get more medications in your IV that will make you go to sleep. You may have a catheter inserted into your bladder after you are asleep, but that last trip to the bathroom helps if your surgeon does not routinely use bladder catheters. Special "boots" may be wrapped around your calves and hooked to a pump to help prevent blood clots from forming in your legs. Your arms will be placed on padded boards at right angles to your body. After you are asleep, the anesthesiologist will insert a breathing tube through which you will get oxygen and anesthetic gases that keep you asleep throughout the surgery. Your chest skin will be washed with one or more antibacterial cleansing solutions, which may be white or pink or brown, and you may see some residue of this when you take your first shower after surgery. The markings that your surgeon made before you went to sleep will be reinforced, possibly with a different color ink. Some surgeons inject the breasts with a dilute solution containing epinephrine that helps to control blood loss.

Breast reduction surgery typically takes from two to four hours, and you will spend another hour or two in the recovery area. You may receive intravenous medications for pain and to prevent nausea. Depending on the medications given, you may have little or no memory of the hours immediately before and after your surgery.

To help you understand your surgeon's decision-making process, it is worth reviewing the goals of breast reduction surgery:

- To improve symptoms
- To decrease the volume and weight of breast tissue without

endangering the blood or nerve supply to the nipple and remaining breast

- To remove excess breast skin
- To elevate the nipple to its proper position in relation to the remaining breast tissue and to the opposite breast
- To create an improved breast shape that will remain stable over time
- To accomplish the above goals with a minimum of scarring

Each operation aims toward these goals, but in fact it is never possible to achieve every goal with 100 percent success for any patient.

The rest of this chapter will give you an overview of the different surgical techniques for breast reduction and will define the medical terms that your surgeon may use during your conversations.

THE OPERATION

Incisions

Most breast reduction patients will have more or less the same operation on both breasts. If your breasts are visibly different in size before surgery, this asymmetry can usually be corrected simply by removing more tissue from the bigger side. When one breast is extremely small compared with the other side, or if one breast is to be reconstructed after cancer surgery (mastectomy), you may need a traditional breast reduction on one side and a completely different operation with different incisions on the other side.

If you are a typical breast reduction patient, you have too much breast skin as well as too much breast tissue, and the excess skin must be removed as part of the operation (Fig. 7–1). Your surgeon will make incisions on your breasts based on where he or she wants the scars to be. In addition, the nipple usually needs to be moved to a higher position (Fig. 7–2). In order to accomplish these two goals—remove excess skin and raise the nipple position—most plastic surgeons make incisions that when closed look like an anchor or an upside-down T (Fig. 7–3). The horizontal limb of the T (or the curve of the anchor) falls in the line under the breast, which is called the inframammary crease.

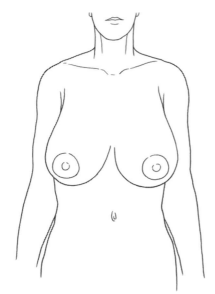

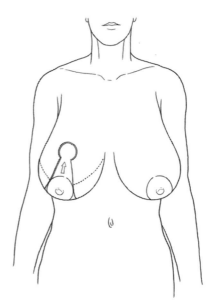

Figure 7-1 Breast reduction patient

Figure 7-2 Typical surgical design

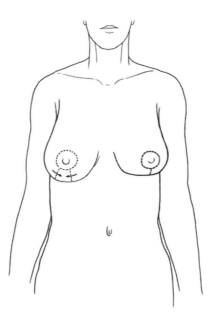

Figure 7-3 Closing the incisions after
the breasts are reduced

The incisions are made in the middle portion of the breast, and all of the lower breast skin, except for the nipple, is removed. The nipple and an appropriate amount of the surrounding darker skin (areola) are usually left attached to underlying breast tissue.

The horizontal incision in the inframammary crease may be short or long, or may be L-shaped instead of T-shaped, depending on your breast size, your overall shape, and your surgeon's choice of procedure. In the 1960s and 1970s, several surgeons in Europe developed designs for breast reduction that do not leave a horizontal scar. These are generally referred to as vertical mammaplasties and are discussed in more detail below.

If you need a relatively small reduction and have good skin tone, you may be a candidate for a procedure that uses more limited incisions, such as a periareolar (incision around the areola) technique or liposuction. One surgeon has recently published his results using a tool similar to that used to shave cartilage during knee arthroscopy. The scope is inserted through a small incision under the breast, and both shaving and internal suturing are done through the scope. This procedure is not widely performed and would be suitable only for very small reductions in young women who have excellent skin elasticity and minimal ptosis (sagging).

Moving the Nipple

LEAVING IT ATTACHED: THE NIPPLE PEDICLE

In many large-breasted women, gravity and breast size conspire to send the nipple below the inframammary crease. This condition is called ptosis (pronounced "toe'-sis"), and correcting ptosis by raising the position of the nipple is one of the major goals of breast reduction surgery. In order for the nipple to survive the move, it either has to be left attached to a healthy amount of breast tissue or it has to be treated like a skin graft. Ideally the nipple is left attached to enough breast tissue that it maintains its blood and nerve supply yet not to so much tissue that the breast remains too large. This tissue attachment is called the **nipple pedicle** and is one of the most important components of any surgical design.

The breast has a rich blood and nerve supply, and the nipple pedicle can be designed from many or multiple segments of the breast. Each design has its proponents and detractors in the medical literature, and most surgeons develop preferences based on experience. Certain designs are more suitable for certain patients. For example, a pedicle that will allow the nipple to be moved up only a few inches is not suitable for a very large-breasted woman whose nipples are at her waist.

The choice of nipple pedicle is usually not obvious to the patient, since the location of the incisions is the same for many pedicle designs. While you need not memorize the technical details of your breast reduction surgery, you should keep a copy of the operative report to give to a future surgeon in the (unlikely) event that you should ever need repeat breast reduction or other major breast surgery.

NIPPLE SKIN GRAFTS

For some patients it simply does not make sense to leave the nipple on a pedicle. In most of these cases, the patient has extremely large and long breasts, and the pedicle would have to be so long and wide that it would be impossible to reduce the breast adequately. As a patient you may also have medical reasons or a smoking history that makes leaving the nipple on a pedicle too risky. Examples of medical conditions that might require your surgeon to perform **free nipple grafting** are a history of previous breast surgery or radiation, diseases that damage blood supply or interfere with healing, any condition that requires you to undergo the shortest possible general anesthesia, and gigantomastia (see Chapter 11). Free nipple grafting means that the nipple and an appropriate amount of areola are completely removed from the breast at the beginning of the operation, to be sewn back on later. Only the skin itself is removed, and all of the milk ducts are cut. The fat is removed from the underside of the nipple graft, and after the breast has been reduced and rebuilt, a circular area of skin the same size as the nipple graft is removed at the new nipple position and the nipple graft sewn in place. The nipple heals as all skin grafts do, by ingrowth of new blood vessels from the underlying tissue. Nipples managed this way have less risk of loss than those left on extremely long pedicles that cannot be relied upon to provide sufficient blood flow all the way to the nipple.

Over time many surgeons have come to realize that free nipple grafting can be avoided in many "borderline" cases by leaving the breasts longer and larger. Substantial weight is still removed, and a nipple on a pedicle can be converted to a free nipple graft during surgery or even immediately after surgery should the nipple blood supply appear questionable. The nipple becomes purple when its blood flow is poor, and since this color change can be virtually impossible to detect in patients with darkly pigmented skin, free nipple grafting may be the preferred option for patients with this skin type who have either long nipple pedicles or the risk factors listed above.

Reducing the Breast

After the breast incisions are made and the nipple pedicle has been separated from the tissue that is to be removed, the surgeon will reduce your breast size. There are limits—removal of too much tissue risks leaving too little blood supply for the nipple pedicle or for the skin and breast tissue that must be preserved for rebuilding the breast. Your surgeon has some leeway as to how much tissue is removed, but your postoperative bra size cannot be absolutely guaranteed. The total tissue removed from each breast is weighed separately and recorded. The breast tissue that has been removed will be sent to the laboratory for routine evaluation under the microscope by the pathologist, a physician who specializes in analyzing tissue. In rare cases the surgeon may come upon an area of breast tissue that does not look normal and will send a piece of the tissue for immediate evaluation, instead of waiting several days for the final laboratory report.

The precise way that the breast is sculpted varies with the technique your surgeon chooses. Each technique has advantages and disadvantages, and some procedures are more "operator dependent" than others. You want to undergo an operation that your surgeon has done many times before.

Detailed descriptions of various techniques are published in the academic literature, but below are short descriptions of the most popular types of operations.

INFERIOR PEDICLE TECHNIQUES

In these procedures the blood and nerve supplies to the nipple are maintained through breast tissue in the lower central portion of the breast. The incisions are typically the inverted-T type. These tech-niques are widely taught in plastic surgery residencies, and over the years continual refinements have maintained them as the most popu-lar techniques for breast reduction.

VERTICAL MAMMAPLASTIES

In the last ten years or so, there has been increasing interest in the United States in breast reduction procedures called vertical mammaplasties. These particular techniques were mainly developed in Europe and do not use a horizontal inframammary incision. The vertical scar extends from the bot-tom of the nipple incision down to and across the inframammary crease and may be puckered for several months (Fig. 7–4). The puckered area usually flattens out as gravity stretches the lower breast skin, but in the meantime the appearance of the breast may be distressing to a patient who is not pre-pared for it. Ten to 20 percent of women having vertical mammaplasties need a future minor surgery under local anesthesia (which may not be cov-ered by insurance) to correct irregularities of the vertical scar. The nipple pedicle itself can be designed vertically (superior pedicle) or horizontally (lateral or medial pedicle). There is a steeper learning curve for surgeons using these techniques, and if you are considering a vertical mammaplasty you should look for a surgeon experienced in the operation.

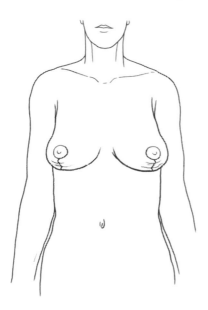

Figure 7-4 Closed incisions after vertical mammaplasties

LIPOSUCTION

Liposuction (suction lipectomy, or SL) is a technique in which tubes attached to a suction machine are inserted through small incisions into fat tissue. The fat is sucked out (aspirated) as needed to contour the area. Special solutions may be injected into the tissue to make it easier to get the fat out. SL is used in two ways for breast reduction. Occasionally, it is used as an additional procedure to help contour the chest, particularly along the sides, during conventional breast reduction. More recently a few surgeons have reported using suction lipectomy, particularly a form called ultrasound-assisted lipoplasty (UAL), to reduce breast size without any major incisions.

Standard suction lipectomy (SL) has the advantages of small incisions and less risk of damage to nipple nerve and blood supply, but the best results are seen in patients with minimal or no ptosis (that is, good nipple position), good skin tone, and mainly fatty (as opposed to dense, nonfat) tissue in the breast. The aesthetic result of SL may be less pleasing if large amounts of tissue are removed without addressing the problem of sagging skin.

UAL is a relatively new liposuction technique in which the breast is injected with a large volume of "wetting solution," and ultrasonic waves and sharp instruments are used to help break up and suck out tissue that cannot easily be removed with conventional suction lipectomy. This technique would seem to lend itself well to removing firm breast tissue. However, one of the disadvantages of using either SL or UAL on the breast is that the removed tissue is severely damaged, and the pathologist looking at it under the microscope cannot determine if the tissue is abnormal. Just as important, the short- and long-term effects of UAL on the breast, in terms of pain, tissue healing, and mammographic monitoring for malignancy, have not been well established. Therefore, as there is limited experience with this technique, if you are considering undergoing UAL for breast reduction you should engage in extensive discussions with your surgeon before proceeding. If you have a strong family history for breast cancer, you probably should have conventional breast reduction surgery so that all removed breast tissue is preserved intact for the pathologist to examine.

Shaping and Closing

Once the reduction portion of the operation is completed, your new breast is shaped. Some surgeons use sutures to help anchor segments of the remaining breast tissue to each other and to the deep chest tissues. A few surgeons use an absorbable mesh, as is used in hernia repairs, to help shape the breast. At this point in the operation, some surgeons prop the still-anesthetized patient into a sitting position in order to assess breast shape before closing the skin incisions. If the breast shape is satisfactory, the incisions are typically closed in two layers. Both dissolvable and removable (surgeons use the terms "absorbable" and "nonabsorbable") sutures, staples, and tape strips may be used. Drains may be inserted to help remove the blood and tissue fluid that leak from the raw surfaces inside the breasts. If drains are used, they usually exit through and are sewn to the corners of the incisions. They are attached to collection devices, such as compressible bulbs, that generate suction to help fluids flow out of the breast rather than pooling inside. Both the choice of closure material and the use of drains is a matter of surgeon training and preference. Studies have shown that patients do equally well with and without drains. In my experience patients who do not have drains have a little more swelling after surgery, but tend to be more comfortable without the tugging of a drain tube. For these reasons I personally prefer not to use drain tubes routinely for breast reduction patients.

Nipple and Areola Size

Many large-breasted women have enlarged areolae, which need to be made smaller during breast reduction surgery so that they look more proportionate on smaller breasts. The nipples themselves are generally left untouched. If a nipple is extremely oversized, it can be made smaller.

Fullness in the Armpit (Axilla)

The breast is shaped like a comet, and the tail is in the armpit. Usually the tail is narrow and tapered, but some women, regardless of breast size, have significant visible bulging of tissue in this area. The bulging may be more obvious on one side than the other. Enlarged breast tissue in the armpit is not only unsightly but, like all breast tissue, can swell and become quite tender during the menstrual cycle because of the normal swelling that accompanies hormone fluctuations. The tail of the breast is not well visualized on a mammogram, and enlargement in this area, although usually benign (not cancerous), may in some situations need to be removed to be sure it does not represent cancer. At the time of breast reduction, excess tissue in the axillary tail can be removed through the main breast incisions, with liposuction or through a separate incision. My experience has been that it is difficult to get a good aesthetic result in many patients without a separate incision in the lower armpit that allows removal of excess skin.

Breast Implants

Hard as it may be to believe, there are a few breast reduction patients who benefit from breast implants. Women who have minimal glandular breast tissue but extensive skin redundancy and sagging, such as after massive weight loss or severe breast atrophy after pregnancy or menopause, tend to have very little breast projection (forward volume) after breast reduction. Before surgery their breasts are long and heavy but very flat, and there isn't enough breast tissue to create projection after the excess skin is removed. Breast implants can create volume and projection to improve the aesthetic result in these patients. If you have decided to add breast implants to your procedure, you are more likely to be given antibiotics and to have drains. If this option is suggested to you, you should discuss the medical considerations and the financial issues in detail in advance. More than likely your insurance company will not pay to have breasts implants inserted. Remember that the insertion of implants will add weight to your chest.

Breast Lift (Mastopexy)

Breast reductions and breast lifts belong to the same family of operations. Some of the same surgical techniques apply to both operations, but breast lifts are designed to deal mainly with sagging, or ptosis. Usually very little breast volume or weight is removed in a breast lift, and in fact some women choose to combine mastopexy with augmentation (inserting breast implants). Since a woman usually wants a breast lift for mainly cosmetic reasons, most mastopexy procedures are designed to limit scars. Mastopexy is not generally covered by insurance plans, which is why most insurance companies require a minimum weight of tissue to be removed during a breast reduction in order for it to qualify for coverage. See Chapter 11 for further discussion of mastopexy.

Anesthesia Options

Most surgeons will recommend that a woman have breast reduction surgery under general anesthesia, described in the beginning of this chapter. General anesthesia is administered by anesthesiologists (physicians) or by specially trained registered nurses (anesthetists).

In select circumstances it is possible to perform breast reduction surgery safely using local anesthesia and intravenous sedation, as long as the anesthesia is provided in a properly accredited facility by appropriately credentialed individuals. In this option the intravenous sedation portion of the anesthesia is begun first. A sedative medication is administered through your IV that will relax you and probably cause you to fall sleep. The dose of sedative is controlled so that you get enough to allow you to sleep, but not so much that you cannot breathe on your own. Next, a local anesthetic (numbing medication) is injected directly into the breasts with a needle. The surgeon performs multiple injections at different locations around each breast in order to obtain adequate anesthesia. The total dose of the local anesthetic medication that is needed can be high, especially if you have large breasts and if liposuction is to be included in the procedure. Local anesthesia with intravenous sedation should be administered only in facilities where the same safeguards and equipment are in place as are required for general anesthesia. Your surgeon will advise you if he or she thinks local anesthesia with sedation is suitable in your case. See Chapter 4 in the section Facility Options for the minimum requirements for a facility offering intravenous sedation.

BLOOD REPLACEMENT

Not that many years ago it was standard practice for breast reduction patients to undergo blood typing and crossmatching in case they needed to receive donor blood. When it became standard practice for patients to donate their own blood (autologous donation), breast reduction patients were sent to the Red Cross station two weeks before surgery. As breast reduction techniques have evolved, this practice is declining. Blood loss during breast reduction surgery may be controlled in a number of ways, including: injecting the breasts with a dilute epi-nephrine solution, which constricts blood vessels; controlling blood pressure during surgery with drugs, especially during the reduction por-tion of the surgery when most of the blood loss occurs; using compres-sion devices or breast tourniquets; and preoperative patient screening and education in order to reduce the risk of excessive bleeding. It is now unusual for a patient to require blood replacement during or after breast reduction surgery.

ANTIBIOTICS

Antibiotics, including intravenous antibiotics and antibiotic washes, are commonly but not universally used during breast reduction surgery. You will likely receive antibiotics if it is part of your surgeon's routine or if you have an increased risk for infection.

DRESSINGS

After breast reduction surgery, you will have dressings that consist of gauze held in place with bandages or a surgical bra. There are many brands of surgical bras, and they are typically built like sports bras with front closures (zipper, hooks, or Velcro) and Velcro shoulder straps that allow easy application in the operating room. If you have drains they will probably be secured to the bra.

ON THE ROAD TO RECOVERY

Your surgery is over. Let the healing begin! Chapter 8 starts in the recovery room.

Chapter 8

The Home Stretch
Recovery

*Y*ou did it! Your surgery is over, and when you wake up from the anesthesia, you will feel lighter. Immediately. Now you are in the home stretch.

BEFORE YOU GO HOME

Recovery Room

After your surgery has been completed and the dressings and bandages or a surgical bra applied, your anesthetic drugs will be stopped. When you are sufficiently awake, your breathing tube will be removed and you will be transferred to the recovery room. You may receive additional medications, such as narcotics for pain, drugs to combat nausea, and antibiotics, in your IV. The nurses will continue to monitor your heart, blood oxygen, and other vital signs. You will stay in the recovery room for one to two hours, and when you are ready for discharge you may go to a "step-down" recovery area if you will be going home that day, or you may go to a regular patient room.

Patient Room

Your stay in the facility may last several hours or overnight. You will continue to receive intravenous fluids, but unless you are nauseated you will be allowed to eat. You can walk and use the bathroom, but ask for help if you feel lightheaded. You will receive medications as needed for pain and nausea. The nurses will monitor your vital signs and will check your surgery site and drains for excessive bleeding. If you do not have drain tubes, there may be some bloody drainage on your dressings. This is to be expected. You may be allowed to shower or bathe before you are discharged, especially if you go home the day after surgery. The nurses should check the color of your nipples and areolae before you go home and notify the surgeon if they are purple, blue, or white. Some nipple bruising and swelling are normal.

The nurses should review your surgeon's instructions with you before you go home and may schedule your next office visit if that hasn't already been done. If you are discharged and do not have an appointment scheduled, you should make one by calling your surgeon's office the next day. Before you go home be sure that you know how to contact your surgeon after hours if you develop an urgent problem.

Length of Stay

If you had a breast reduction in the 1970s, you likely would have stayed in the hospital for two or three days. Beginning in the early 1980s, cost-containment efforts ignited an explosion in the volume of outpatient surgery, and many procedures, including breast reduction, were converted to outpatient or extended outpatient (often called short-stay or twenty-three hour stay) status. As it turns out, patients have done just as well with shorter stays as they used to do with longer hospitalizations. Now, a breast reduction patient is likely to stay in the hospital or surgery center for just under twenty-four hours. This is true for most of my patients, many of whom benefit from the overnight hospitalization for pain and nausea control. However, my younger patients (especially those without small children) often go home the day of surgery, and I have even had at least one hardy patient insist on going straight home from the recovery room. Shorter stays cost less, and I encourage patients who are paying for surgery out of pocket to plan to go home the day of surgery if possible.

Some plastic surgeons perform breast reduction surgery in their office operating suites, which may or may not have the capability for patients to stay overnight. If a patient cannot go home after surgery for unanticipated medical reasons, she will be transferred to a local hospital. You should find out in advance what your surgeon's protocol is for this situation.

If you have preexisting medical problems, such as lung or significant heart disease, or any other condition that requires you to be observed closely after surgery, your doctor will recommend that you have surgery in a hospital and perhaps be admitted as a regular inpatient for a day or two.

Serious complications are extremely rare after breast reduction surgery, but if they do develop, you will of course need to be kept in the hospital as long as is necessary to treat the problem.

AFTER YOU GO HOME

For the first few days you will have some pain and possibly some nausea and vomiting. It is a good idea to have someone stay with you for at least twenty-four hours after surgery. After that, arrange for someone to check on you frequently for a day or two. Remember, you should not be driving during this stage of your recovery.

Pain Control

Pain after breast reduction surgery is to be expected but should not be excruciating. Some patients have very little pain, and I have had a few take no pain medication at all. The typical patient, however, will need pain control for one to three weeks after surgery. In the hospital I order intravenous and oral narcotics for my breast reduction patients, and they receive a prescription for oral narcotics to use at home. You should take your prescribed pain medication according to the instructions on the bottle. Keep in mind that narcotics and general anesthetics can impair your judgment. Do not make important decisions or sign legal contracts for at least twenty-four hours after the surgery. You will probably not need narcotics after the first week or two after surgery, and you should not drive or operate any kind of machinery until you have stopped taking narcotics.

You may have a sore throat from the breathing tube. Throat lozenges usually help, and this discomfort rarely lasts more than a day or so.

Some women have chronic shoulder problems that limit their shoulder mobility. These patients may notice aggravation of their shoulder pain immediately after surgery because of the positioning required during the operation. If you experience this problem, you can take your usual pain medications or anti-inflammatories. Applying heat and/or ice to the affected shoulder(s) may also help. This problem usually improves within a few days.

Some patients cannot tolerate narcotics for a number of reasons: allergy, nausea, hallucinations, headaches, constipation, or simply an unpleasant feeling of lightheadedness or disorientation. If you have trouble with narcotic pain medications or if you no longer wish to take them, use ice packs and over-the-counter medicines like acetaminophen and ibuprofen. If you prefer acetaminophen (for example, Tylenol), I recommend the extra-strength version taken according to the instructions on the bottle. If you want to take ibuprofen (for example, Motrin, Nuprin, or Advil), ask your doctor if you can take prescription-level doses (600 to 800 milligrams every six to eight hours). You can alternate doses of acetaminophen and ibuprofen, since they are chemically unrelated. Do not take more than the recommended dosage of either drug within any twenty-four-hour period.

Ice packs are very helpful for controlling pain. Get out your little bags of frozen peas (see Chapter 6). You can tuck them into your bra as needed and refreeze them when they thaw. Throw them away when you do not need them anymore—do not eat!

Most patients do not need to take pain medications on a regular basis after several weeks. You may have breast swelling and pain during your first menstrual period after surgery, and sexual stimulation may cause your breasts to swell and ache during the first month or so. You may feel a generalized discomfort in your breasts for a few weeks and may experience occasional shooting pains in the breast area for months, but these will become less frequent as time passes and usually stop altogether before the end of the first year after surgery.

Nausea Control

General anesthesia can cause nausea and vomiting, and some patients are more susceptible to these problems than others. Many anesthetic drugs bind to fat, so overweight patients are especially prone to prolonged nausea or lightheadedness after general anesthesia. Newer anesthetic drugs, such as propofol, have lessened this problem, and anesthesiologists routinely give intravenous drugs during surgery to help prevent subsequent nausea and vomiting. Even so, some patients have nausea with or without vomiting for a day or two after surgery. If narcotics cause you nausea, you may do better with nonnarcotic pain medicines, such as ibuprofen and acetaminophen. For nausea that persists, drugs that may help include Zofran, Compazine, Phenergan, and Tigan (rectal suppository). Rarely, a patient may have unrelenting vomiting, which can cause dehydration. If your mouth feels dry and you become increasingly lightheaded after multiple episodes of vomiting, or if you simply are too nauseated to take any fluids for a day, you should call your doctor, who will likely recommend that you go to the emergency room. Many times patients can receive intravenous fluids in the emergency room and return home without the need for admission to the hospital.

Antibiotics

Not all plastic surgeons routinely order antibiotics for breast reduction patients. Patients who are at increased risk for infection are those with current rashes or infections of the breast skin, overweight patients and others with a high percentage of fat in their breasts, and patients with poor personal hygiene. Patients in these higher-risk categories are more likely to receive antibiotics for surgery. Other patients with special risk factors, such as mitral valve prolapse (especially if symptomatic), and implanted foreign bodies like heart valves and artificial joints may require antibiotics during the period immediately before and after surgery.

Washing, Wound Care, and Dressings

Every surgeon has preferences for wound care. My patients usually do not have drains, and I allow them to shower starting the day after surgery. I do not recommend baths for wound care, although it is okay to soak in the tub up to your waist.

For wound care I instruct my patients to do the following: Wear your surgical bra at all times except in the shower. Every day remove your bra and dressings (soak the pads off in the shower if they stick to your incisions), and wash your breasts and incisions with antibacterial soap and water. Pat your incisions dry. If you develop any open areas within the incisions, apply an antibiotic ointment (for example, Neosporin, Bacitracin, or generic triple antibiotic) to these areas after cleaning. You can buy these ointments over the counter. Apply clean dressings and a clean bra. For the dressings you can use menstrual and nursing pads or gauze. If you have a lot of drainage, you should change the pads or gauze more frequently or add extra padding during the day. If you use an antibiotic ointment and develop an itchy rash, stop using the ointment and notify your surgeon. Hypersensitivity reactions to these ointments are very common, especially after they have been used for a week or more. In this situation I prescribe Bactroban or generic mupirocin, which is a prescription antibiotic ointment unrelated to those listed above and is usually very well tolerated. If your skin feels dry, you can use any type of moisturizer as long as you do not get it near your incisions.

Wash and air-dry your bras daily. If the bra that you received at the surgery facility is too tight, you can wear any sports bra that closes in the front. *Never* continue to wear a bra that is uncomfortably tight.

Drainage and Drains

Breast reduction surgery creates large, raw surfaces inside the breasts, and these raw surfaces ooze blood and serum for several days. Active bleeding stops almost immediately after surgery, but serum mixed with blood that has collected inside the breasts will be present for weeks. Most of these fluids will be absorbed as healing progresses. Some fluids will come out of the breast through drain tubes or through your incisions. The drainage will look like pure blood the first day. After that its appearance will evolve from thin pink to thin clear yellow.

It may be your surgeon's routine to use drains and to leave them in place for as little as a day or as long as a week. If your drains are attached to collection devices and will stay in place for more than a day, you or your caregiver helper may have to empty the collection devices and record the amount of drainage. This is not a difficult task, and you will receive instructions on how to do it before you go home.

Do not be alarmed by small amounts of crusting on your incisions or by a pink or yellow clear drainage on your dressings. These findings may persist for several weeks or until your wounds are completely healed.

A (usually minor) complication called fat necrosis (see Chapter 10) can result in wound drainage days or weeks after surgery. You might have a low-grade fever with no obvious source, or you may develop increased pain and a red, tender area in the involved breast. Depending on the circumstances, if your surgeon thinks that you may have some fat necrosis, he or she may decide either to watch and wait or to drain the breast surgically in the office or in the operating room. If you are "watching and waiting," be aware that the liquefied fat, which looks like pus, may drain suddenly and profusely through one of your incisions. Put extra absorbent pads into your bra so that you are prepared if this should occur. Even though the sudden drainage can be frightening to the patient, it usually leads to dramatic relief of the fever and discomfort.

Smoking

If you managed to quit smoking before surgery, you deserve a big "Congratulations!" Keep it up. In order to protect your nipples, it is critical that you do not smoke for *at least* the first week after surgery and preferably for far longer. Remember: This is a risk factor that *you* can control.

Diet and Activity Level

Breast reduction surgery is basically a skin operation. No body cavities, muscles, bones, or joints are involved. Therefore, you can eat according to your usual diet, and you need not and should not stay in bed all day. Walking is encouraged: It keeps your strength up, lowers the risk of blood clots in your legs, and helps prevent constipation (which can be a problem if you are taking narcotics for pain). But don't overdo it, especially during the first few days. Sleep in any position that is comfortable, but you will probably find yourself sleeping on your back for a while. Many women are not accustomed to sleeping on their backs and complain about this aspect of recovery more than about the pain! Try using extra pillows to support your breasts so that you can sleep partially on your side.

I recommend that patients do not drive until a week after surgery *and* when they are no longer using narcotics. You should avoid moderate to heavy lifting for approximately one month after surgery and avoid strenuous exercise and sports (for example, tennis, swimming, golf, aerobics) for at least six weeks and longer if your incisions are not healed. You can get in the shower, but you should not expose any open wounds to a swimming pool, lake, or other areas of potentially contaminated water. Sex should be avoided for at least two weeks. (As noted above, sexual activity may cause uncomfortable breast swelling for several weeks longer.)

While you may not have much pain after a week or two, you must remember that your body is putting a lot of energy into healing your breasts, and you will not have your usual stamina for about six weeks. Take it very easy for the first two weeks, and then *gradually* increase your activity level until you are back to your normal routine. If you plan to start a new exercise program, be sure that your incisions are completely healed. Start slowly. Check with your surgeon if you are unsure how active you can be, especially if you have had any delays in healing. Check with your regular doctor before embarking on *any* new, strenuous exercise regimen. Before you start exercising, make sure that you wear a good sports bra. See Chapter 3 for what to look for in a sports bra.

Regular Medications

For the most part, you should resume your regular medications the day after surgery. If you take insulin or blood thinners, check with your doctors regarding the timing and dosage of these medications.

Alcohol

Alcohol can contribute to excessive bleeding and should be avoided immediately after surgery. You also should not drink alcohol while you are taking narcotic pain medications.

WHEN TO CALL THE DOCTOR

Since you have read this book you know what to expect after surgery, and you will probably not need to call your surgeon other than to make a routine appointment. However, you *should* call your surgeon if you think that you are having problems. The following are the most common potential problems for which you should notify your surgeon (see Chapter 10 for more information on these and other potential complications):

FEVER

Fever over 100° F in the first twenty-four hours after breast reduction surgery is common and usually turns out to be caused by fat necrosis (see Chapter 10). Even small areas of fat necrosis can cause fever. There are other potential causes of fever, especially after the first twenty-four hours, and your surgeon may start you on antibiotics if you are not already taking them.

BLEEDING

You may be having excessive bleeding if, for example, you have any of the following: noticeable enlargement of one or both breasts; increasing pain, especially if only on one side; continuous bloody drainage from the incisions that requires you to change your dressings multiple times in the space of a few hours; or enough blood in your drains that you have to empty them considerably more frequently than you were instructed to do. Notify your surgeon *immediately* if you are at all concerned that you may be actively bleeding.

FOUL ODOR AND DRAINAGE

Foul odor is caused by infection and/or dead tissue and is usually accompanied by fever and increasing pain. There may also be cloudy fluid or matter draining from your incisions. Profuse, nonbloody drainage two to six weeks after surgery is frequently a manifestation of fat necrosis. If this occurs (often in the middle of the night), do not panic. Clean yourself up, put some extra absorbent padding in your bra, and call your surgeon in the morning.

BLUE NIPPLE

Immediately after surgery your nipples will be bruised in areas, but they should still be basically pink. Light-skinned women can do this quick "capillary refill" test of nipple and areola blood supply: Gently press your finger on the nipple and areola skin. When you lift your finger, the color in the spot where you pressed should look paler for a split second and then rapidly return to pink. If your nipples are purple or blue or gray, or if the color does not return (or returns very slowly) after pressing, *notify your surgeon immediately*. Patients with very dark skin generally cannot use this test of nipple blood supply. For any patient, however, if your nipple seems unexpectedly cool to the touch, especially when compared with the other nipple, call your surgeon. These tests do not apply to patients who have had free nipple grafting.

PROLONGED VOMITING OR INABILITY TO TOLERATE ANY LIQUIDS FOR TWENTY-FOUR HOURS

It is important to avoid dehydration after surgery, so be sure to notify your surgeon if you cannot take in or retain fluids by mouth, if your mouth and tongue feel dry, or if you are urinating only small volumes of concentrated (dark) urine.

Doctor's Office Visits

The number and frequency of your follow-up visits will depend on your surgeon's routine and on your progress. If you have drains, you may be seen within the first few days for drain removal. Typically, patients will be seen in the surgeon's office about one week after surgery and once or twice more in the early healing phase. During these visits the drains (if you have them) and the stitches or staples will be removed, and your breasts will be examined to assess the progress of healing. Some surgeons recommend long-term application of topical ointments or silicone pads to the scars in the hope of reducing scar thickening. Your surgeon may ask you to return to the office in six to twelve months and possibly yearly thereafter, to reassess your breast shape.

Ask for a copy of your operative report. (It may be several weeks after surgery before the report becomes available.) If you should ever need a repeat breast reduction or other major breast surgery, your future surgeon will welcome detailed information about prior disruption of the nipple blood supply.

What to Expect From your Breasts

COLOR

Immediately after surgery your body starts to build new blood vessels and to increase flow through the old blood vessels in your breasts in order to bring in oxygen and other nutrients for healing. Particularly if you have fair skin, you will be aware of this increased blood flow by the pinkish color and increased warmth of your breast skin. If you do not have a fever and do not feel that your pain level is increasing, you can relax about these color and temperature changes. They are normal parts of the healing process and will subside over a period of weeks to months. You also will have substantial bruising. At first the bruising will be red or purple, and over the next few weeks it will change to green and yellow before fading. These color changes represent the normal breakdown of blood that leaked into your skin during and after surgery. Just as your skin changes color, the drainage on your dressings may change from red to yellow. Clear yellow drainage is not pus and does not indicate infection.

SHAPE

Right after surgery your breasts will *not* look like what you signed up for! *This is normal.* In fact, breast reduction operations are designed with the understanding that gravity is a fact of life and the expectation that your skin will stretch.

If your surgeon performed the common inferior pedicle operation or a related procedure, your breasts will look square right after surgery. As the swelling goes down and your lower breast skin stretches, a more natural, rounded breast shape will develop. This reshaping process starts early after surgery, but is not complete for at least six months.

If your surgeon performed a vertical mammaplasty, your breasts may at first look too cone-shaped and may have puckered incisions running from the nipples or below to the lower breast creases. Again, it will take several months for these irregularities to improve.

If you are overweight and have excess skin and fat along the sides of your chest behind your breasts, this excess may be relatively unchanged or may even feel somewhat more prominent because of swelling and because your breasts are no longer heavy enough to pull the skin and fat along the sides of your chest forward and down.

Events that occur during the healing process will affect each breast differently. There will always be more bruising, swelling, or pain on one side compared with the other.

SIZE

Expect your breast size to decrease slightly as healing progresses and the swelling subsides. It may take a few months for all of the swelling to disappear.

INCISIONS

Complete healing of your incisions may take as little as two weeks or as long as six weeks, depending on many factors, and during that time small amounts of drainage or bleeding are common. Certain areas of the incisions are prone to delayed healing, such as under the breasts where the limbs of the "T" incisions meet. Occasionally, a patient will develop a reaction to the internal dissolvable sutures, causing small areas of prolonged drainage. These healing problems are easily managed with good wound care and are usually resolved within a short time. Your incisions are healed well enough for you to get into a swimming pool when you have no further drainage or crusts along your scars. Scar strength takes longer to develop, which is why you should avoid heavy lifting and strenuous activities, including actual swimming, during the four to six weeks after surgery.

SCARS

All skin incisions heal by forming scar tissue. Scar tissue varies in appearance from patient to patient (for genetic reasons) and from one part of the body to another. Typically, breast scars are red, raised, and firm for months after surgery. They may itch or be irritated by your bras. You may experience occasional shooting pains near the scars, especially under your breasts and near your armpits, during the first year after surgery. These pains are part of the healing process and subside in time.

NIPPLES

One or both nipples may feel numb after surgery. This is a common occurrence after breast reduction and may be temporary or permanent. Temporary numbness can be the result of swelling or bruised nerves and usually subsides within weeks to months. Permanent nipple numbness occurs when nerve fibers are cut during surgery. Permanent nipple numbness can occur after any type of breast reduction operation. Some women, in contrast, notice increased nipple sensitivity after breast reduction, and the reasons for this are not fully understood. Annoying nipple hypersensitivity usually subsides within a few months.

If your nipples were removed completely and sewn back on (free nipple grafting), they will almost certainly be numb and permanently flattened after surgery. Partial loss of nipple color (depigmentation) can occur in any breast reduction patient and may be temporary or permanent. Free nipple grafts almost always depigment and become permanently pink or splotchy in color. This is particularly noticeable in dark-skinned patients.

If your nipples were inverted before surgery, they will still be inverted after breast reduction. Drainage from the nipple ducts after surgery is uncommon but can occur. The drainage may be clear or bloody (usually brown, like old blood). Always report any nipple duct drainage to your surgeon. If at all possible, try to identify which duct is draining (squeeze the nipple gently to see if you can express a drop of liquid).

CHEST WALL PAIN

For most women, chest wall pain gets better after breast reduction surgery. However, different types of chest wall pain and tenderness can develop that are direct consequences of the surgery. First, sharp shooting pains along the sides of the chest and breast are common. These pains often last for months, but become less frequent and less severe over time. They are probably related to irritation of the nerves along the sides of the breast during removal of breast tissue in this area. Second, an occasional patient will develop a blood clot in a vein on the surface of her chest (see Chapter 10). This can lead to a painful lump under the skin that may persist for several months.

Buying Bras

You will find that sports bras fit better than do regular bras during the first four to six months after breast reduction surgery. Some patients may be able to wear their old bras (and fit into them, for a change!). Avoid bras with underwires for at least six weeks. When your scars are soft and your breast shape is starting to look more rounded, you can start shopping for regular bras. Look for bras with stiff fabric support instead of underwires. If you have trouble finding a bra that fits comfortably, go to a specialty shop that employs professional fitters (often a shop that caters to larger women and to mastectomy patients) rather than to a store that only sells sexy lingerie.

Pregnancy

If you get pregnant after having breast reduction surgery, your breasts will go through the same changes that they would have gone through if you hadn't had surgery (see Chapter 2). The difference, of course, is that there will be less of your breasts to change. Breasts start to swell and become tender very early in pregnancy. I recommend that patients avoid getting pregnant after breast reduction until their breasts have had a chance to heal well, which usually takes at least four to six weeks.

FEARS AND ANXIETIES

Immediately after surgery you may experience euphoria. It's over! What a relief! After you come back to earth, you will feel a sense of well-being, which over time becomes increased self-confidence and improved self-esteem. Sounds great, doesn't it? So what's the problem? Between the immediate sense of excitement and relief and the later improvement in self-esteem can lie a swamp of unexpected feelings. These feelings may range from disappointment to outright depression. The fact is that every woman who has a breast reduction has to develop a new body image. A woman's body image is formed by her psyche and will not necessarily reflect the physical condition of her body. Creation of your new body image will be both a conscious and an unconscious process and will not occur overnight or even within a few weeks. It takes *months*, and while it is happening you will almost certainly have some anxieties. *This is normal.* Here are some common fears and unexpected feelings:

- "My breasts are gone."
- "My breasts are still too big."
- "My nipples are going to fall off."
- "Something is missing."
- "I'm not me anymore."
- "I feel unprotected."
- "I see large-breasted women and I envy them."

You can have the same feelings that someone might have after losing any visible body part. An occasional woman may even develop a prolonged depression after surgery.

Breast reduction surgery may alter your feelings about your sexuality, and it will take some time for your new sexual identity to evolve. How breast reduction affects your sexual psyche depends in large part on how old you were when your breasts became large. Women who developed early in adolescence often have more complicated sexual anxieties about breast reduction than do women who experienced breast enlargement later in life. Regardless of their developmental history, however, most women adjust to the surgical changes in the appearance of their breasts within the first year.

Few women talk to their surgeons about these psychological issues, and, frankly, some surgeons may not be sensitive to or even aware of them. A great source of support can be another woman who has had breast reduction surgery. If you do not know one, ask your surgeon to connect you with a former patient. In the meantime take comfort in knowing that having anxieties or a sense of mourning are normal and even predictable. These feelings may come and go but eventually will subside. YOU ARE NOT CRAZY.

Also, remember that even though anxieties are common, the vast majority of women who have undergone breast reduction surgery will tell you that the permanent relief of physical symptoms far outweighs the temporary psychological distress. Few women ultimately regret their choice to have the surgery.

Chapter 9

Satisfaction
Expectations and Results

*I*magine for a moment that a year has passed since your breast reduction surgery. Was it worth it? Do you look and feel the way that you expected to? I hope in this chapter to give you a good sense of what to expect so that your results will mirror as much as possible your expectations.

Plastic surgeons have noticed for decades how happy breast reduction patients are after surgery, even though these women have had surgery that put scars on their breasts. The reason for such a high satisfaction rate is that the surgery relieves multiple debilitating symptoms and improves the overall health status of almost every patient. The results of numerous recent scientific studies of breast reduction patients, which have been undertaken in order to prove the benefits of the surgery to insurance companies and employer benefits specialists, have proven that breast reduction surgery leads to predictable improvements in a long list of symptoms, physical abnormalities, psychological distress, activity level, and quality of life. Breast reduction surgery may also provide direct and indirect economic benefits to both patients and their employers.

SYMPTOMS

When the researchers analyzed the results of the BRAVO study (see Chapter 5), for which they had interviewed hundreds of women, they were amazed to discover that women with symptomatic breast enlargement have far more pain than doctors have ever realized. What was not surprising was that their study finally provided plenty of medical evidence to show that breast reduction surgery helps relieve women of multiple symptoms, including:

- back pain
- neck pain
- shoulder pain
- headaches
- arm and hand pain and numbness
- skin irritation and rashes (intertrigo)
- shortness of breath

Deanna: "I do not have that nagging back pain that I used to have every single day. I sleep so much more comfortably. It's incredible. I just feel so good."

Lyn: "I used to get migraines at least once or twice a week. I have not had a single headache since my surgery [six weeks earlier]."

Amy: "Everything has gone away. The back pain, the shoulder pain, the numbness in my hands. I did not get any rashes last summer. The surgery was the best thing I have ever done for myself."

Most women experience significant or complete relief of a variety of types of pain and numbness. Skin rashes and irritation are usually completely eliminated. A woman's sensation of shortness of breath may disappear. In fact, you will be the rare patient if you do not experience significant or complete relief of many of your physical complaints.

The study results also showed that the improvement in symptoms experienced by breast reduction patients is independent of their body shape, body weight, bra cup size, or the amount of breast tissue that was removed at surgery. In other words, if you are overweight you are just as likely to benefit from breast reduction surgery as is a woman who is not overweight. If you have severe symptoms and are larger-busted than average but not huge, removing a relatively small amount of breast weight can be just as helpful as would removing a larger amount of weight from another woman's breasts.

The studies documented that the improvements in symptoms after breast reduction surgery persist for years, regardless of whether a woman's weight changes. In fact, even if you gain weight after surgery you probably will not have to go back to a bigger bra cup size.

When the researchers looked closely at the symptoms experienced by women with heavy breasts, they found that *women having breast reduction surgery felt better not only in comparison with how they felt before surgery, but actually felt as good or better than did a group of women of the same age who did not have heavy breasts!*

If you have symptoms due to an underlying medical problem, you may experience more limited improvement. Even so, you may find that your pain requires much less medication for control.

PHYSICAL EFFECTS

With smaller and lighter breasts your upper body is able to function more normally. You should notice:

- Improved posture
- Increased back and shoulder muscle strength
- Improved lung function

Carmen: "I don't slouch anymore! It's incredible to have that heavy burden finally lifted off my shoulders. Now I can lift my grandkids without suffering for days afterward."

Joyce: "I can finally breathe easier. It's difficult to breathe when you have two watermelons on top of your chest."

Your posture and muscle strength have been disturbed for a long time and will not become normal overnight. However, most postural disturbances not related to an uncorrected anatomic abnormality (such as scoliosis) are reversible. In Chapter 3 you will find some useful stretches and exercises. If you need more help or if you find that your shifted center of gravity is causing new pain, ask your surgeon to prescribe physical therapy. Usually, a short course of therapy and instruction does the trick.

Shoulder grooving is one of the few physical effects of excess breast weight that may be permanent, especially in older patients who have had to support heavy breasts for many years.

Lung function is rarely abnormal in otherwise healthy women with large breasts, but even so, testing after breast reduction surgery often shows improvement in breathing capacity. Even without formal testing you may notice such an improvement simply by feeling less short of breath.

YOUR BREASTS

Immediately after surgery your breasts will have an odd shape, as discussed in Chapter 8. By four months their shape will start to look more natural, and by six to nine months the shape will be fairly stable. After one year you will probably not notice any significant changes in your breast size or shape unless you undergo a major change in hormone levels, such as occurs during pregnancy, menopause, or hormone therapy. If you are under the age of eighteen and your breast size had not stabilized for a year or two before you had surgery, you may experience further breast enlargement (see Chapter 11).

One of a plastic surgeon's goals during breast reduction surgery is to sculpt breasts that ultimately will have improved shape. As the patient, you hope for a breast shape that is pleasing and natural. How your breasts look after surgery is determined by their unique characteristics before surgery, the procedure chosen, and whether or not there are any complications during the healing process. In general, you can expect:

- Smaller breasts that sit higher on your chest.
- Reasonably symmetrical breast size, shape, and nipple position.
- Breasts that are about the same width they were before surgery.

- Visible scars.
- Breasts that may not project forward (best noted on side views) as much as you would like, especially if they were composed mainly of excess skin before surgery.

Breast reduction surgery corrects significant asymmetries of breast volume. Perfect symmetry of breast shape, size, and nipple position is not possible for several reasons. First, no woman is perfectly symmetrical before surgery, and the reasons for asymmetry may not lie in the breasts themselves. No woman has symmetrical shoulder girdles and chest wall structures. Muscles, bones, joints, and all related attachments can be significantly more developed on one side or may simply be different from one side to the other. Second, plastic surgeons can weigh only what they take off, not what they leave behind, and have to assess visually (while she is still asleep on the operating table) if a patient's breasts are reasonably symmetrical. Third, it is humanly impossible to perform the identical procedure on two breasts, especially since they are on opposite sides of the body.

When a complication of breast reduction surgery (such as bleeding, infection, and fat necrosis) develops, it frequently affects only one breast. Occurrence of a complication can result in long-term, although not necessarily severe, breast asymmetry.

Of the many factors that affect the final shape of your breasts, there are several over which you and your surgeon have no control, such as skin type, skin elasticity, and genetically determined healing characteristics. You may also have limited control over any coexisting medical conditions.

Surgeons choose the surgical procedures with which they are most comfortable and that they feel are most suitable for their patients. Experienced surgeons have a better feel for the design aspects of this surgery than do those who have performed it infrequently, but no surgeon can promise perfection.

Nipple/Areola Color, Contour, and Sensitivity

Most women having breast reduction surgery will undergo a nipple pedicle procedure, in which the nipple/areola complex is moved up on the breast but left attached to underlying breast tissue. In this type of operation, the color of the nipple and areola is maintained, unless there are healing problems. The areola is usually made smaller and more round in shape. Nipple sensitivity may be unchanged, decreased, or increased. Many large-breasted women do not have much nipple sensitivity, but others are very concerned that loss of nipple sensation will reduce the erotic pleasure that they derive from their breasts. All breast reduction procedures remove tissue that may contain tiny nerves to the nipple area, and some patients will lose some or all nipple sensitivity on one or both sides. Some sensation may return over time, but the degree and timing of improvement cannot be predicted. For unidentified reasons, some women experience increased nipple sensitivity after surgery. It is impossible to predict for any given patient how much nipple sensitivity she will have after surgery.

Patients who undergo free nipple grafting almost always lose nipple sensitivity, nipple erection, and nipple and areola pigmentation. Pigment changes are particularly noticeable in patients with dark skin, in whom the nipple/areola complex may become pink or splotchy. In some patients, a certain amount of pigmentation will return during the first year or more. Splotchiness is the result of an incomplete return of pigmentation. If you have experienced bothersome pigment changes, you can ask your surgeon about tattooing for pigment restoration. However, tattoo pigments are prone to fading over time.

The nipple itself, in contrast to the areola, is usually left unaltered during surgery, even though some patients may have preexisting nipple irregularities. Nipple inversion is not usually corrected during breast reduction surgery in order to minimize disruption of nipple blood supply. Overly large nipples can be safely reduced in size during breast reduction surgery or at a later time.

Chest Contour

Some women have large breasts that are further accentuated by lower rib flaring. Rib flaring refers to the permanent expansion of the lower rib cage that often develops during pregnancy, especially in short-waisted women. Breast reduction surgery does not correct rib flaring.

Heaviness along the sides of the chest wall can be the result of excess fat or redundant skin or both. This contour may be improved if some of the excess fat was removed during surgery. Bulging due to excess inelastic skin will be improved only if your surgeon extended the skin incision, and thus your scar, along the side of your chest toward your back. If full-ness along the sides of your chest is still a problem when you get ready to buy new bras, go to a shop that specializes in fitting larger women. Chest wall fat does decrease with weight loss.

Scars

Naturally, you would prefer not to have scars, but if you are like the vast majority of women who have had breast reduction surgery you will judge your scars to be acceptable, especially considering the benefits of getting the weight off. Breast reduction scars are per-manent and always visible to some degree (Fig. 9–1). They may itch, especially along the segments rubbed by your bra, but the itching will decrease and eventually go away in most cases. Your scars will flatten and fade and may also widen as they mature. Scar widening seems to happen more often in patients

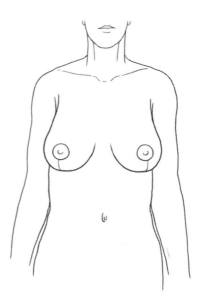

Figure 9-1 Final scars

who are prone to stretch marks, and it is especially common in the por-tions of the scars most subject to gravity, such as the area above the areolae. Fine-line scars are rare on breast skin. You should expect some difference in color (lighter or darker) and texture between the scars and the surrounding skin.

Scarring is a particular concern for women of color, who may worry about forming keloids. If keloids are going to develop, they will do so within the first few months after surgery. Fortunately, keloids are very rare in breast reduction surgery and are very unlikely to develop in a patient who does not have a keloid history. Problem scars—hypertrophic scars and keloids—are discussed further in Chapter 10.

Breastfeeding

Approximately half of women who attempt to breastfeed after breast reduction surgery (nipple pedicle procedures only) are able to do so successfully. A significant number of women who have never had breast surgery cannot nurse for a variety of reasons, so it is difficult to predict breastfeeding success for any particular patient. A woman who has had breast reduction surgery with free nipple grafts will produce milk postpartum, but will not be able to nurse because her milk ducts have been cut. As with all postpartum women who do not nurse, milk production stops, and any milk that has been produced will be absorbed by the breast. A woman who strongly desires to nurse future children may wish to delay breast reduction surgery until she has completed childbearing.

Mammograms

Regular mammograms (breast X-rays) should be part of every woman's health care, in order to maximize the chances of detecting breast cancers early. Breast reduction surgery results in changes that are visible on a mammogram, including altered breast contour, distortion of the internal breast architecture, scarring, fat necrosis, asymmetrical densities, and the late appearance of coarse microcalcifications (calcium deposits). Except for the calcifications, these findings are usually most prominent early after surgery and improve over time. Calcifications, on the other hand, are frequently not seen until the second or third year after surgery. Even so, coarse calcifications are the most common type of calcification and are not the type of calcium deposits often seen in breast cancers.

I recommend that a woman postpone having a mammogram after breast reduction surgery for approximately one year, even if she is "due" for one earlier. Her breasts will be tender for quite a long time after surgery, and the compression required for a good mammogram can be quite painful if performed early in the healing process. When you are ready to have your first mammogram after surgery, be sure that the radiologist reading the X-ray knows that you have had breast reduction surgery. If the radiologist is uncertain about any findings on your mammogram, one of three things is likely to happen. First, you may be asked to return for additional X-rays, which will help the radiologist evaluate the questionable area further. Second, you may be asked to have the next mammogram of the breast in question in six months instead of the usual one year, so that the area of concern can be checked for change. Third, it may be recommended that you have a biopsy done of an area of concern. Most of the time, changes on mammograms after breast reduction surgery can be evaluated adequately without requiring biopsy.

PSYCHOLOGICAL RESULTS

Even though insurance companies do not value the psychological distress suffered by women with large breasts, women and their surgeons know that the psychological benefits of breast reduction surgery can be just as liberating as the physical benefits. It has been repeatedly documented that after surgery women experience a dramatic increase in self-image and self-esteem. You are much less likely to think of yourself as overweight, even though your weight hasn't changed that much. You will likely be less preoccupied with how much you weigh. Your outlook on life will be sunnier. You will be ready to go places and try things that you wouldn't have dreamed of doing before your surgery. You will look forward to social events much more than you did in the past. Now that you can buy clothes to fit, your back isn't bothering you so much, and people don't stare at your chest anymore, you will feel more relaxed in public.

> *Tina:* "This surgery changed my life. My self-esteem is so high. I'm so happy. I can't thank you enough."

> *Jackie:* "I am finally in proportion. My top is the same size as my bottom! Before, even when I was thin my top was at least two sizes bigger than my pants, so I could never buy two-piece outfits or dresses."

Linda: "I never bought new shirts when I was pregnant, since I already had huge ones to cover my breasts. I couldn't wait to throw those tents away."

Geri: "At restaurants I always had to eat in an awkward manner because my chest stuck out so far. I would lean forward and stretch out my neck in an uncomfortable way so that food wouldn't drip on my 'shelf.' Even after surgery I still ate that way because I was so used to it. Then one day I went to a restaurant, actually sat in a booth, and had four inches between my chest and the edge of the table! I was amazed!"

Suzanne: "It made me feel sad when I was eight-and-a-half months pregnant and nobody could tell because my breasts were so big. Now I feel like my shape is normal."

Tammy: "I couldn't wait to go shopping after surgery and buy a bra that wasn't beige or white. And a bathing suit! I hadn't worn one in six years."

Marlene: "I can really hug my kids close now instead of feeling like they're a foot away."

Gina: "It's hard to explain how HAPPY I am. I have wanted this surgery since I was eleven years old."

Occasionally, there is a downside to this "new lease on life" experience. Your family and friends may have higher expectations for you and may say things like: "Now get on that diet!" "Find new friends!" "Get straight A's!" You need to keep your perspective. Your life *will* be better in many ways, but in your own time and not all at once.

ACTIVITY LEVEL

Women who undergo breast reduction surgery often experience a dramatic increase in their overall activity level. Suddenly they are able to perform their jobs better and to accomplish tasks, including housework and other chores, which they simply could not manage before surgery. Mothers and grandmothers are thrilled to be able to play games with their children and grandchildren. These women have increased exercise tolerance and more energy for all activities, which leads to even more participation. An impressive result of the research studies was that before surgery nearly all of the women were unable to participate in sports of any kind, whereas after surgery nearly all could participate in sports. It is now a well-established fact that people can improve their health and longevity simply by increasing their activity level.

> *Delores:* "The surgery has changed my life. It's the best decision I have ever made. My knees don't hurt, my back pain is gone, and I don't get out of breath when I walk. I love to walk! Thanks to you, Doctor, I have a second chance to make my life longer and healthier."

QUALITY OF LIFE

Breast reduction surgery can provide you with relief of many of your daily frustrations. For example:

- You can store your pain pills in the medicine cabinet instead of on the counter for easy access. The studies have shown that women who have had the surgery are much less likely to use medications such as pain pills, anti-inflammatories, and muscle relaxants. In fact, the rate of use of these medications drops to a level no higher than normal.

- You can also put away the medicated creams that you have been using on the rashes under and between your breasts. Once your breasts no longer rest on your upper abdomen, you will not have the combination of moisture and lack of air circulation that allows bacteria and yeast to thrive in your breast creases. If you do not need to wear underwire bras, you will experience complete relief of the chronic irritation under your breasts, even in warm weather.

- You can go shopping! Nothing gives a breast reduction patient more pleasure than going to a store and buying not only bras but bathing suits, shirts, and jackets off the rack that fit, perhaps for the first time in her adult life.

- You can recharge your love life. Naturally, this is a complicated issue, but in the medical studies a third of women reported improvement in their intimate relationships, and very few (less than 5 percent) reported worsening. Chapter 11 discusses this topic in more detail.

ECONOMIC BENEFITS

It is very difficult to measure productivity changes in the diverse group of women that participates in a study, but every individual knows how the surgery has affected her life and job performance. It seems obvious that a woman who suffers from back and neck pain is more likely to stick with or apply for a high-paying job that requires lifting or other strenuous physical activity if she is able to achieve permanent relief of her pain. Anecdotally, many women have told me how much easier their jobs have become since their surgery.

Chapter 10
Complications

$\mathcal{A}$ll surgeries can have complications, and a breast reduction is more prone to complications when there is a large volume of fat in the breast or when the nipple has to be moved a long distance. Women who are overweight also have a higher complication rate, even though there is no evidence that preoperative weight loss reduces this risk. In any case, most complications are minor and can be managed without further surgery or hospitalization. This chapter will review the most common potential early complications, both local (related to the surgery site itself) and systemic (affecting the body as a whole and which could develop after any major surgery performed with general anesthesia). I will also discuss late complications, which are significant problems that affect the long-term appearance of the breasts.

EARLY BREAST COMPLICATIONS

Infection

WOUND

Any surgical incision can become infected. A wound infection is detected by the presence of redness, swelling, increased pain, and sometimes pus draining from a portion of the incision. A true wound infection is usually treated with oral antibiotics and sometimes with suture removal. Redness and mild irritation confined to the area directly around stitches or staples usually represent a skin reaction to the suture material rather than infection. Antibiotic ointments can also cause redness and rashes and should be discontinued or a different ointment used if a rash develops.

True wound infections are uncommon in breast reduction surgery. More often we see an isolated area of wound breakdown, which can result from infection around a buried stitch or from a point of tension in an incision. This type of problem is almost always successfully treated with local wound care. I recommend twice a day cleansing with an antibacterial soap followed by the application of an antibiotic ointment and a clean, absorbent pad.

ABSCESS

An abscess is a collection of infected fluid (pus) and dead tissue inside the surgery site. In the breast an abscess usually declares itself by an area of redness, swelling, and increased pain. The patient often has a fever. The key to treatment of an abscess is drainage, which in some cases can be performed in the surgeon's office. Drainage of a deep abscess is more extensive surgery that usually requires a return to the operating room. Occasionally, an abscess will drain on its own through an incision or even through the skin. However drainage is accomplished, most surgeons will also prescribe antibiotics to treat any remaining infection.

Breasts are particularly prone to another problem called fat necrosis, which can look very much like an abscess. Fat necrosis is discussed below.

GENERALIZED BREAST INFECTION

Overall breast redness, increasing swelling, increasing pain, and fever could indicate a serious infection of the entire breast. This is an extremely rare but very serious problem and should be evaluated by a doctor immediately.

Fat Necrosis

The term "fat necrosis" refers to fat that does not survive an injury (such as surgery). Some women have a lot of fat in their breasts, while others have relatively little. Women with fatty breasts have a higher likelihood of fat necrosis after breast surgery. Fat necrosis is a particular problem in breast reduction surgery because extensive incisions are made through fat tissue that already has poor blood supply compared with other body tissues. Fat that has borderline blood supply will look normal to the surgeon during the operation, but after the breast incisions are closed and swelling begins, what was borderline blood supply becomes inadequate blood supply. The affected fat tissue becomes inflamed and eventually dies. The fat globules themselves turn into a yellow, greasy liquid. Liquefied fat irritates surrounding tissues, which causes more inflammation and sets the stage for infection of the dead tissue.

A patient with fat necrosis will develop an area of pain, redness, and swelling in the breast. Often only one breast is affected. Sometimes the liquefied fat will drain out through an incision. The drainage can be sudden and dramatic, but also signals the beginning of improvement. Once drainage begins, the pain and inflammation usually start to subside. The drainage is usually a cloudy, greasy yellow liquid but can also be green or brown, especially if there is infection or blood mixed with it. Drainage may persist for days or even weeks but tends to lessen over time. I encourage patients who develop an area of fat necrosis to put absorptive pads with waterproof backing (for example, menstrual pads) into their bras.

In rare cases liquefied fat cannot find its way out through an incision and will present as a soft, red spot in the middle of the breast. In this situation the surgeon may need to make an opening in the skin to allow the liquefied fat to come out. Fat necrosis may be associated with a fever, which usually subsides as soon as the liquefied fat is drained. Antibiotics may be prescribed for fat necrosis in case bacterial infection is also present.

Small areas of fat necrosis may never drain, but instead leave firm areas inside the breast, particularly in the region of the nipple and the nipple pedicle. These hard areas eventually soften over a long period, usually many months.

If significant fat necrosis occurs in one breast and not in the other, there may be permanent visible asymmetry of the breasts. Further surgery may be needed to improve symmetry. Fat necrosis may also cause irregularities that are visible in mammograms. Most of the time these changes can be monitored with serial X-rays, but occasionally a breast biopsy of the irregular area will be recommended to rule out cancer.

Skin Separation (Wound Dehiscence)

If the breast incisions are closed under tension, the skin edges can separate as breast swelling increases in the first few days or later, after the sutures or staple are removed. Wound separation is called dehiscence and is most common under the breast at the T junction. Infection, fluid and blood collections, and fat necrosis can also create openings in the incisions at points of drainage. Small areas of wound separation can be managed with dressing changes and wound care. Larger areas may require further surgery. Fortunately, minor degrees of skin separation usually heal well without any negative effect on the final appearance of the scar.

Skin Necrosis

Skin necrosis means loss of skin due to poor blood supply or severe infection. Major skin loss is rare after breast reduction surgery. Factors that can be responsible for significant skin necrosis include surgery on a patient with a heavy smoking history or a history of previous irradiation of the breast (such as for breast cancer); development of a large blood collection (hematoma) inside the breast after surgery; and technical aspects of the surgical procedure (such as the creation of thin skin flaps or closure of the skin under tension).

Bleeding/Hematoma/Seroma

Excessive bleeding is not common after breast reduction. If bleeding does occur, it may be the result of one or two leaking blood vessels or of a previously undiagnosed bleeding problem. Plastic surgeons have developed numerous ways to reduce blood loss during breast reduction surgery. However, the operation does create extensive raw surfaces inside the breasts, and these raw surfaces ooze blood. All patients will have significant bruising of the breasts after surgery. An occasional patient will develop a collection of blood inside the breast that can result in prolonged swelling, pain, and firmness. This collection of blood is called a hematoma. Small hematomas will be absorbed in time and do not require treatment. Larger hematomas require drainage, either in the office or in the operating room. Hematomas can develop both in patients who have drains placed during the breast reduction operation and those who do not have drains. Some patients develop seromas, which are collections of fluid (serum) that oozes from the cut surfaces inside the breast after the bleeding has stopped. Seromas are frequently absorbed by the body without requiring treatment but occasionally have to be drained. Often this can be performed in the surgeon's office.

Generalized persistent bleeding after surgery may indicate a bleeding disorder, which more than likely would be suspected during the operation. Surgeons strive to identify patients with potential bleeding disorders before surgery, but if a bleeding problem is suspected during or after the operation it must be evaluated and treated aggressively. Certain drugs impair blood clotting, and you should avoid them before surgery (see Chapter 6). Pregnancy and breastfeeding dramatically increase the blood supply of the breasts, and elective breast surgery should be delayed for several months in recently pregnant and nursing women (also see Chapter 6).

Nipple Loss

Nipple loss refers to failure of the entire nipple and areola to survive. Fortunately, this is an uncommon occurrence after breast reduction surgery. The risk of this complication increases with the length of the nipple pedicle: that is, the distance that the nipple must be moved up on the chest. Nipple loss can also result from postoperative obstruction of breast blood supply by, for example, an excessively tight bra. Nipple loss could be virtually eliminated if all patients had free nipple grafts, but a nipple left attached to a pedicle looks and feels more natural. Marginal necrosis (loss limited to the edge) of the areola skin is fairly common and is treated locally, just like any minor incision problem. Free nipple grafts and nipples with borderline blood supply may "peel," much like a bad sunburn. This is called superficial desquamation, which refers to loss of just the top few layers of skin cells. Ultimately, these nipple-areola complexes usually heal very well.

If a nipple-areola complex is congested after surgery, it will look purple. If it appears salvageable, the surgeon may prescribe topical nitroglycerin ointment to increase its blood flow. Nitroglycerin is a vasodilator, which means that it opens up blood vessels. This drug is also used by patients who have pain due to heart disease (angina). The amount of nitroglycerin ointment needed to improve blood flow in a nipple-areola complex is very small, but even so this medication may cause headaches in some women. If the survival of a nipple remains questionable despite use of nitroglycerin, urgent surgery may be required. Many times the surgeon will have to remove the nipple and replace it as a free graft, but occasionally the nipple can be maintained on its pedicle after pressure on the pedicle is reduced. It is sometimes possible to achieve adequate relief of pressure and improve blood flow to the nipple by removing the sutures, repositioning the pedicle, and possibly further reducing the breast in order to give the pedicle more room inside the breast. Naturally, further reduction of breast size may result in some breast asymmetry if the opposite breast is not made smaller as well.

If the nipple blood supply is inadequate for too long, the nipple tissues will undergo irreversible damage and will not be salvageable, even after conversion to a free nipple graft. Therefore, it is imperative that you notify your surgeon immediately if you notice any duskiness or purplish discoloration to the entire nipple and areola or if you notice loss of capillary refill (see Chapter 8 for a description of a simple test to check capillary refill). If the nipple and areola do not survive, a portion of the underlying pedicle will also likely be lost. Dead tissue may be removed in the office or in the operating room as it separates from healthy tissue. The end result will be a somewhat smaller breast without a nipple. Nipple reconstruction can be performed once scars have matured, which takes many months. Some asymmetry between the two breasts is likely.

Chest Cords

An occasional patient will develop a painful cord (superficial phlebitis) under the skin in her lower chest after breast reduction surgery. This cord represents an inflamed vein, which may have a clot in it. The cause may be the surgical bra or the surgery itself. In any case, treatment consists of warm packs and pain medication. The cord may take weeks or months to resolve completely.

Galactorrhea (Milk Drainage)

Women who were pregnant or who breastfed within a year prior to breast reduction surgery may have residual breast milk inside their milk ducts. These patients may have milky drainage from the nipple or through the incisions for a short time after surgery. Rarely, a woman who has not been pregnant recently may have milk drainage, and she may require a hormone and pituitary gland evaluation.

Unanticipated Breast Cancer

I think it must be every woman's nightmare that her plastic surgeon will open her breasts and find cancer. In fact, this event rarely occurs. Less than 1 percent of breast reduction patients have a breast cancer diagnosed during surgery. Keep in mind that all breast reduction patients are screened ahead of time. They have breast examinations before surgery, which include checking for signs of cancer, and most women will have a mammogram before surgery. Even so, a cancer is occasionally encountered during a breast reduction. If the surgeon finds a suspicious area, a piece of tissue will be sent to the laboratory for immediate examination (called frozen section). If cancer is diagnosed, the incisions will be closed and the surgery terminated. The patient will be referred to the appropriate specialists for further evaluation and treatment.

Sometimes a cancer is not obvious to the plastic surgeon and is discovered by the pathologist performing the routine examination of the removed breast tissue. In that situation, the patient will also be referred to the appropriate specialists.

EARLY SYSTEMIC COMPLICATIONS

Anesthesia Complications

General anesthesia and local anesthesia with sedation (conscious sedation) are administered uneventfully millions of times a year to help patients undergo surgery comfortably. General anesthesia should only be given by well-trained physicians (anesthesiologists) and nurses (anesthetists). Some plastic surgeons use local anesthesia with intravenous sedation for breast reduction surgery. Most hospitals require surgeons wishing to provide this type of anesthesia without an anesthesiologist present to be specifically credentialed to administer conscious sedation. If your surgery is to be performed outside a traditional hospital setting (such as in an office suite), ask about the facility's accreditation and the credentials of the personnel who will be administering your anesthesia and monitoring you during and after surgery (see Chapter 4).

Anesthetic complications are uncommon, and in healthy patients they are rare. Complications that can occur range from minor (nausea or sore throat from the breathing tube) to serious (heart attack or seizure) to devastating (stroke or death). This chapter does not cover every potential complication of surgery, but does discuss the most common. I have no qualms about recommending surgery with general anesthesia to any patient for whom it is medically appropriate. Since you probably will not meet your anesthesiologist prior to the day of surgery, feel free to ask your surgeon about the providers of anesthesia at the institution where the surgery will be performed.

LUNGS

Atelectasis

Atelectasis refers to the collapse of small air sacs in the lungs and is fairly common in patients who undergo general anesthesia. Atelectasis is one of the common causes of fever in the first twenty-four hours after a general anesthesia, but is much less common in young, healthy patients. Prevention and treatment consist of deep breathing and early ambulation after surgery.

Pneumonia

Untreated atelectasis or a preexisting respiratory problem can lead to pneumonia, which is an infection of the lung. Pneumonia is rare after breast reduction surgery.

HEART PROBLEMS

Cardiac complications during surgery are rare in healthy patients, and even women with known heart disease can often undergo general anesthesia if they have been properly evaluated and prepared. Even so, heart rhythm irregularities (arrhythmias) or inadequate blood flow to the heart (ischemia) can occur during anesthesia. Anesthesiologists are trained to handle these problems if they occur. A patient who experiences a significant cardiac "event" during surgery may be transferred to a cardiac care unit afterward and evaluated by a heart specialist (cardiologist).

BLOOD CLOTS

• Deep Venous Thrombosis (DVT)

A blood clot in a deep leg vein is a serious problem, and if you have a history of DVT you are at risk for recurrence. Deep vein clots cause leg swelling, but more important, they can break off and lodge in the lungs. Other factors that increase your risk of DVT and pulmonary embolism (see below) are the use of contraceptives, hormone replacement, a family history of thrombosis or embolism, a genetic disposition to blood clotting disorders, and any swelling or other signs of poor vein function in your legs.

• Pulmonary Embolism (PE)

Blood clots that enter the heart and get lodged in the vessels of your lungs are called pulmonary emboli. Pulmonary emboli can be fatal. If you have any history of DVT or PE, you must notify your surgeon before surgery. Preventive measures can be taken to minimize your risk for either complication. The treatment of DVT and PE usually includes blood thinners, but as a general rule patients who are on blood thinners should not undergo major elective surgery such as breast reduction unless the blood thinners can be stopped temporarily. A patient with a history of DVT or PE who cannot be on blood thinners or must stop taking them may be a candidate for the insertion of a filter into the large vein going to the heart (inferior vena cava) that prevents leg clots from reaching the lungs.

URINARY RETENTION/BLADDER INFECTION

Some patients have difficulty emptying their bladders after general anesthesia, especially if large volumes of intravenous fluids are given. Temporary urinary retention is treated by the brief insertion of a bladder catheter. Rarely, women with persistent problems require a longer-term catheter or appropriate medications.

A woman may develop a bladder infection if she has difficulty emptying her bladder or if she requires a catheter. I do not routinely order bladder catheters for my patients in order to minimize the risk of causing a bladder infection. However, if your surgeon anticipates that your surgery will take more than three hours, you may need a catheter both to avoid excessive bladder distention and to allow the anesthesiologist to monitor your fluid balance. Bladder infections are treated with antibiotics and oral fluids. Notify your surgeon in advance if you are prone to bladder-emptying problems or infections.

LATE BREAST COMPLICATIONS

Skin Pigment Alterations

The scars after breast reduction surgery will always be a different color from that of the surrounding skin, regardless of a woman's natural skin type. Pigment loss is a particular issue for women of color. Partial pigment loss may occur in nipples maintained on pedicles, especially if there was marginal necrosis (see section above on Nipple Loss). Loss of pigment in the nipple and areola is nearly universal in free nipple grafts and may be permanent. Nipple tattooing to restore color is an option for women who are bothered by the pigment changes.

Problem Scars

Occasionally, a woman will develop breast scars that remain red, raised, and painful. These **hypertrophic scars** are most common in young, usually fair-skinned patients. However, they can occur in patients of all skin types. Hypertrophic scars usually improve over time, but there are a number of treatments that sometimes improve those scars that are particularly bothersome. Surgical revision is usually not helpful, although if a hypertrophic scar is the result of infection or delayed healing, surgical excision and closure may be all that is needed. Other treatment options include locally injected steroid medication, steroid tape or cream, silicone sheeting, pressure garments, laser treatments, and radiotherapy.

Keloid scars are a concern for all patients, but more so for women of color. They are more common in younger patients. Keloids are thick, cauliflower-like scars that grow beyond the borders of the original incision. Keloids are related to but are not the same as the more common raised red hypertrophic scars that remain confined to the incisions. Like hypertrophic scars, keloids may be painful or itchy. Keloids can be described as a scar in which the healing process is turned "on" and never turned "off." True keloids should never be treated with surgery alone, since they may recur in a more severe form. Injected steroids and/or radiation therapy may be helpful alone or in combination with surgical excision. Keloids are difficult to treat and may be impossible to control. Fortunately, they rarely develop after breast reduction surgery. A patient with a personal or family history of keloids needs to discuss this problem in detail with her surgeon, who can help her estimate her risk for developing keloid scars after breast reduction.

After surgery the weight of the breast pulls on the scars under the breast. Some wound separation and prolonged healing in this area is common. Often this delayed healing has little effect on long-term scar appearance, but occasionally the scar under the breast will widen excessively and may result in prominent discoloration in this area. It may be possible for the surgeon to revise this scar to improve its appearance, but most patients are not overly concerned about scarring in this relatively hidden location.

Sometimes scars are visible beyond the borders of the breast. Occasionally, this problem can be improved with an additional minor surgical procedure to reorient the visible portion of the scar.

Cysts

Several surgical designs for breast reduction surgery require the surgeon to remove barely more than the thin top (epidermal) layer from a portion of otherwise retained breast skin, most notably on the nipple pedicle. This process is called deepithelialization. Very thin deepithelialization leaves tiny islands of epidermis inside the breast, and sometimes these islands form cysts similar to the skin cysts people can develop from acne or similar problems. These cysts can become infected or can rupture and cause irritation and inflammation in the breast. Occasionally, antibiotics and surgical drainage are required for treatment.

Asymmetry

Mild asymmetries of size, shape, or nipple position between the breasts are common, even normal (see Chapter 9). If a woman develops a complication such as fat necrosis in one breast, she may ultimately have a major size or shape discrepancy between her breasts. Further surgery will likely be required to correct this problem, but is usually delayed until healing is complete and tissues have softened.

Shape Problems

No surgeon can guarantee a perfect result or a particular cup size, and you may very well notice some features of your new breasts that you wish were different. This does not mean that you have had a complication. However, there are some results that are not desirable and which usually can be corrected with additional surgery.

- **Size**
Your breasts may be much bigger or much smaller (two or more cup sizes different) than you expected. Perhaps there were technical or medical reasons why the surgeon could not achieve your goal, or perhaps you developed a complication, such as fat necrosis, that resulted in one or both breasts being too small. Perhaps you and your surgeon did not have a clear understanding of your size goal. Breasts that are still too big after the swelling is gone can be further reduced surgically. Breasts that are too small usually require the insertion of breast implants to increase volume.

- **Shape**
Shape irregularities can result from complications, such as fat necrosis. Undesirable contours can also develop as a consequence of the effects of gravity on the breast, especially on the nipple pedicle, particularly in patients with poor skin elasticity. Excess breast tissue, fat, or skin is fairly common at the ends of the horizontal incision (called "dog ears") or along the vertical incision in vertical mammaplasties. Many of these problems can be corrected surgically if they do not resolve within six months to a year.

Nipple/Areola Size, Shape, Contour, or Position Problems

If the areola diameters are persistently unequal after surgery, they can usually be equalized by making the larger side smaller. If a nipple is severely off center on the areola (keep in mind that some asymmetry is common even in breasts that have never undergone surgery), a minor surgery can improve or correct the problem. Minor surgery can also correct less common problems, such as distortion or puffiness of the portion of the areola. Some women have huge areolae before surgery, and it is not always possible to remove all of the excess pigmented skin. Those patients will be left with some residual pigmentation along the vertical scar between the nipple and the crease under the breast. For a patient who is bothered by this persistent pigmentation, it may be possible to remove the remaining darker skin once the breast scars have matured.

The nipple is in a good position when it looks right in relation to the bulk of the breast, to the crease under the breast, and to the opposite nipple. If a nipple is too high in relation to the breast and to the crease, it can be lowered surgically but usually at the expense of leaving a new scar in the breast skin above the nipple. If a nipple is in good position in relation to the crease, but the breast tissue has sunk below it (known as "bottoming out"), it may be possible to correct this problem through the original incisions. Asymmetrical positioning of the nipples may require further surgery, although keep in mind that this problem may in fact not be a complication at all, but rather is the result of asymmetry between the two sides of the chest wall and the shoulders. Chest asymmetry, if it exists, would have been present before surgery, but may not have been noticed by the patient when her breasts were bigger and her nipples were lower on her chest.

Recurrent Breast Enlargement

This is an undesirable event but not a complication of the surgery per se. Recurrent enlargement should be distinguished from persistent excessive size, in which the breasts are still too big after surgery.

Recurrent enlargement is usually the result of persistent hormone stimulation, either during puberty, from pregnancy, or from the use of hormones in medications (birth control pills, hormone replacement therapy, or in the treatment of certain types of cancer).

Need for Further Surgery

There are two time periods after breast reduction when you might need more surgery. First, you might need further surgery in the early healing phase if you develop a major complication. For example, one or both nipples might need conversion to a free nipple graft, you might have significant bleeding, or you might develop an area of infection or fat necrosis that has to be surgically drained. Fortunately, these serious events are uncommon, and most complications are less severe and can be treated without a return to the operating room.

Second, you may have significant irregularities of your breast contour or a major discrepancy in breast size that requires another surgery to correct. Surgeries to correct these kinds of problems are usually postponed for six months to a year after the initial breast reduction, until complete scar maturation has occurred and final breast contour can be assessed.

Secondary procedures may be performed under local anesthesia or may require another general anesthesia. Your insurance may not cover the second procedure, and you should determine your financial obligations before proceeding with any nonurgent surgery. You should also find out what your activity limitations will be after the second surgery. In most cases, restrictions will be minimal.

The choice whether to have more surgery to correct a contour irregularity is yours. The irregularity may bother your surgeon more than it bothers you. By the same token, you may be bothered by an irregularity that your surgeon does not feel can or should be corrected. In that situation you should feel free to seek a second opinion from another plastic surgeon. From a strictly medical standpoint, there is no "deadline" before which you need to have further surgery, although there does usually need to be a period of six months to a year after the original surgery and healing before additional surgery should be performed.

The Dissatisfied Patient

Dozens of studies have shown that the vast majority of breast reduction patients are happy that they had the surgery and would choose to do it again. What about the minority? In general, several observations can be made:

- Patients who are dissatisfied are often those for whom the cosmetic aspects of the surgery are more important than the relief of symptoms.
- For every dissatisfied patient there are many others who are pleased with the same physical outcome.
- Dissatisfaction is often not the result of a serious complication.
- Patients who do experience a serious complication do not necessarily become dissatisfied with the end results of surgery, even if the results are not optimal.
- Dissatisfaction is often the end result of poor communication between the patient and the surgeon.
- Dissatisfaction is more likely to develop in a patient who is not educated before surgery as to what outcomes she can reasonably expect.
- A patient with unrealistic expectations is more likely to be dissatisfied with the outcome of her surgery. For example, a woman with a very specific mental image of exactly how her breasts should look is likely to be disappointed after surgery, especially if she has not fully recognized her desires or has not been able to communicate them to her surgeon.

No one wants to go through major surgery and be dissatisfied with the results. Chapter 9 discusses expectations and results at length. In order to maximize your chances for a satisfying result keep these points in mind:

- Do not expect surgery to alter your life radically, even though your life *is* likely to improve.
- Your result will not be perfect.
- You will have visible scars.
- No surgeon can guarantee a cup size. If you have a preference, tell your surgeon in advance.
- Complications are not uncommon in breast reduction surgery, but most of them are minor and do not substantially detract from the long-term outcome.

- Undesirable results often can be improved with additional surgery.
- If you are unhappy with your results, *talk to your surgeon* about it. Do not expect him or her to read your mind. Most surgeons want nothing more than for you to be a happy patient. In some cases your surgeon may not be able to offer you the solution you are seeking. In that case I recommend that you seek a second opinion from another plastic surgeon. Your surgeon may offer this option to you. Neither you nor your surgeon should take personal offense at this suggestion, since having another opinion is often extremely helpful and reassuring.

Chapter 11

Special Concerns

BREAST REDUCTION DURING ADOLESCENCE

Dramatic breast enlargement during adolescence, especially for the youngest girls, can be psychologically devastating. The physical changes of adolescence are one of this life stage's major developmental stresses, and girls who are destined to be large-breasted usually begin breast development early. Early breast enlargement can overshadow all of the other insecurities and anxieties of early adolescence and can adversely affect a young girl's ability to cope with sexual relationships and win peer group acceptance.

❋ My youngest patient, Shauna, was twelve years old when she came to see me. She was very thin but was already wearing a DDD cup. None of her classmates were nearly as developed as she was, and she was not emotionally prepared for the attention that her breasts were getting, especially from older boys and men. During our consultation her mother had to do most of the talking, since all Shauna could manage was to look at the floor and wipe the tears from her eyes. The problem from my standpoint was that she wasn't finished growing, and her breast size had not stabilized.

If breast reduction surgery for girls like Shauna is not delayed, there is an extremely high chance that they will need a second surgery. Repeat surgery carries higher risks (see page 178), so plastic surgeons try to avoid operating on teenagers too early. Typically, a plastic surgeon wants a girl's breast size to have been stable at least for one and preferably for two years before she has a breast reduction. Exceptions may be made for severe psychological distress, severe physical symptoms, or true gigantomastia (see page 173).

Girls who develop large breasts during adolescence can have the same constellation of symptoms that adult women have, although the girls' physical deformities may be limited to the postural abnormalities that arise as they try to hide their breasts. When I see a teenager with multiple symptoms and physical complaints and who has perhaps given up sports or other activities because of her breast size, I know that I am looking at someone who is facing an adult life of increasing pain, weight gain, decreased activity level, and so on in a vicious cycle, unless something changes. Breast reduction surgery can make a dramatic difference for these girls, as long as they understand the risks and benefits. Studies have shown that of all the age groups that make up the plastic surgery population, adolescents receive some of the greatest psychological benefits. As a general rule, teenagers are better able than adults to adjust their body images after surgery (see Chapters 1 and 8).

When I evaluate a young woman for breast reduction surgery, I make sure that we discuss each of the following issues, all of which are discussed in more detail elsewhere in this book.

Scars

Young women are very body conscious and do not want scars. A few patients will be candidates for minimal scar breast reduction procedures (see Chapter 8), but very large-breasted girls will need traditional operations that result in more visible scars.

Nipple Sensation

Some large-breasted girls have very little nipple sensation, and for some of them, nipple sensation may improve after breast reduction.

However, women of all ages must understand that permanently diminished or lost nipple sensation is a well-known but unpredictable side effect of breast reduction surgery.

Future Pregnancy and Breastfeeding

Young women need to know that their breast size and shape will change with future pregnancies. There is also no way to predict if they will be able to breastfeed after breast reduction. Concerns about breastfeeding may cause some young women to postpone having breast reduction surgery.

Future Breast Examinations and Mammograms

Breast reduction surgery causes scarring inside the breasts that will alter the appearance of breast tissue on a mammogram (breast X-ray). I do not order preoperative or postoperative mammograms on patients under the age of thirty unless there is a special indication to do so. Teenagers undergoing breast reduction surgery should be aware that scarring from surgery will impact future breast exams, and I encourage them to learn and practice regular breast self-examinations (see Appendix B).

Continued Breast Enlargement

As mentioned earlier, breast reduction surgery should be delayed if at all possible until breast size has been stable for a minimum of one to two years. If a teenager is severely symptomatic, and she and her family and the surgeon have agreed to proceed with surgery, she must understand that her breasts may continue to enlarge and that she may even need another surgery with greater risk in the future.

GIGANTOMASTIA AND EMERGENCY BREAST REDUCTION

Gigantomastia (also known as juvenile virginal hypertrophy of the breast) is a rare condition in which a patient, often a young girl who has just started menstruating, develops rapid, massive breast enlargement. Occasionally, the condition may develop in a pregnant woman. Gigantomastia usually affects both breasts and in some cases may be a familial trait. If massive enlargement occurs in only one breast, other possible causes need to be considered.

Gigantomastia almost never gets better on its own. It can be painful, and the growth of breast tissue can be so rapid that the blood supply to the breast becomes insufficient. When that occurs, large portions of the breast tissue can die.

The treatment of gigantomastia is radical breast reduction, usually with free nipple grafting. Surgery may be required on an emergency basis to prevent complications, but recurrence of the problem after surgery is common, especially in pregnant women or when surgery is performed on a young girl before her breast size has stabilized. In those cases repeat surgery may be required. In some cases total mastectomy (amputation of the breast) is required to control the process. Some physicians have treated these patients with surgery and tamoxifen, a drug used in the treatment of breast cancer, which may help control breast overgrowth.

True gigantomastia is caused by an abnormal response of breast tissue to the female hormone estrogen. In the other more common and usually long-standing type of massive breast enlargement, a woman develops huge breasts—cup size J or K, for example—over many years because she has generous breast tissue coupled with extremely stretchy skin. Her breasts may hang to her hips, but some surgeons do not believe this condition should be called gigantomastia because it behaves differently from hormone-induced rapid breast enlargement. Both types of massive breast enlargement can cause severe physical and psychological symptoms, but only the woman with the chronic "stretched skin" type can anticipate the same degree of permanent symptom relief from surgery that is experienced by most breast reduction patients.

BREAST REDUCTION FOR WOMEN WITH EATING DISORDERS

There is plenty of evidence that many women develop dysfunctional eating habits in response to their excessive breast size. As discussed in

Chapter 1, women have admitted to keeping themselves overweight purposely in order to deemphasize their breasts. These women are often in a constant battle with their weight, swinging between onerous diets and anxious overeating in an attempt to normalize their body proportions. Therefore, it is not surprising that some young women with overly large breasts develop pathological eating disorders like anorexia nervosa and bulimia nervosa. Eating disorders have traditionally been characterized by dangerous weight control behavior due to extreme dissatisfaction with body image. Therapy is usually focused on managing the underlying psychological conflicts, while little attention has been paid to what may be a very real and treatable physical problem.

Bulimia nervosa is the eating disorder most commonly associated with large-breasted women. Bulimia is characterized by repeated bouts of binge eating followed by inappropriate "make up for it" behavior, such as self-induced vomiting; improper use of medications like diet pills, diuretics, and laxatives; fasting; and excessive exercise to prevent weight gain. If a woman loses substantial weight, she may well notice a slight decrease in breast size. Teenagers and young women readily use this evidence to justify continuing their dangerous eating habits. Eating disorders and the associated psychological disturbances can become so severe in adolescents that breast reduction surgery may have to be considered at an earlier age than is usually considered ideal.

Several studies have been published in which researchers interviewed women with bulimia nervosa whose large breast size seemed to be contributing to their eating disorders. A study from the University of Rochester showed that breast reduction surgery in carefully selected patients with eating disorders was very helpful not only in the treatment of symptoms related to excessive breast size but also in the management of the eating disorder. These improvements persisted, and after ten years none of the women who were reinterviewed reported any eating disorder behaviors.

A candidate for breast reduction surgery who is known or suspected to have an eating disorder should (1) be actively attending an eating disorder program; (2) understand how her large breasts are affecting her physical, psychological, and social functioning; (3) have realistic expectations for the physical, psychological, and social results of surgery; and (4) have a good support system of family and friends.

The surgeon should be made aware of her eating disorder at the initial consultation and should work closely with the patient's psychiatrist or therapist if surgery is planned. Surgery alone, without appropriate psychotherapy, is not appropriate for a woman with a severe eating disorder, and surgery may not be appropriate at all for some women. For women with an eating disorder diagnosis, it is crucial that psychiatric care be initiated and maintained throughout the period of surgical management and beyond.

PREGNANCY AND BREASTFEEDING AFTER BREAST REDUCTION

Women who become pregnant after having breast reduction surgery will experience the usual pregnancy-related changes in their breasts. These changes vary in degree from woman to woman. During and after pregnancy, breasts may enlarge, droop, shrink, or change very little. Obviously, a woman who has had a prior breast reduction will have less breast tissue to go through these changes. Women who have had breast reduction surgery may or may not be able to breastfeed successfully, which is also true of women who have never had breast surgery. The exception to this is women who have breast reduction surgery with free nipple grafting: None of these women will be able to nurse because all of their milk ducts have been completely detached from the nipples.

MAMMOGRAMS AND CANCER SCREENING BEFORE AND AFTER BREAST REDUCTION

Women who have had breast reduction surgery should undergo the same monitoring for breast cancer before and after surgery that all women of the same age and risk group should. (See Appendix B for instructions on how to do breast self-examination.)

Women should have mammograms regularly, according to the current recommendations by the American Cancer Society. Those guidelines, as updated in May 2003, include:

- Screening mammogram every year for women age forty and older
- Breast examination by a health professional every three years for

women ages twenty to thirty-nine and yearly for women age forty and over

- Breast self-examination monthly by all women starting at age twenty
- Possible additional testing, such as ultrasound or MRI, for any woman in a high-risk category for breast cancer

I also recommend preoperative mammograms for all patients age thirty and over, and for any patient with a strong family history of or other high-risk factors for breast cancer. Postoperative mammograms are ordered as described in Chapter 9.

Breast reduction does not cause breast cancer and may in fact reduce a woman's chances of developing breast cancer. A recent analysis of six studies involving 32,000 women suggests that breast reduction surgery may lower a woman's risk of developing cancer by 50 percent to 70 percent. Breast reduction surgery may in fact make breast cancer easier to diagnose, since adequate mammograms are difficult to perform on extremely large breasts. A pathologist should evaluate the tissue that is removed during surgery, and if the surgeon encounters any suspicious areas during the surgery, those areas should be sampled and sent to the pathology laboratory for immediate evaluation (frozen section). Rarely, a breast cancer may be diagnosed in a breast reduction specimen, and the patient will need to be further evaluated and treated appropriately for the type of cancer.

Unfortunately, there are currently no universally accepted recommendations for whether and when women younger than forty who are planning to have breast reduction surgery should have mammograms. Most surgeons would agree that women under the age of forty with a personal or family history of breast cancer need to have mammograms before and after surgery. Breast cancer is rare in women under thirty, so a common protocol for breast reduction patients without high-risk factors is to require those over thirty to have a recent mammogram *before* surgery. Some plastic surgeons also recommend that these patients get a baseline mammogram about one year *after* breast reduction to document changes related to surgery. Under normal circumstances these would be the only mammograms that most patients would get until they reach the age of forty, at which time current American Cancer Society standards would apply.

BREAST REDUCTION IN THE BREAST CANCER PATIENT

Breast reduction may play a role in the treatment of breast cancer. The operative design of a breast reduction may be used for a mastectomy (although the nipple may not be preserved) or a lumpectomy (in which the nipple may be preserved). Breast reduction surgery may be appropriate for the breast without cancer in order to achieve symmetry and/or to reduce the lopsided physical discomfort of having a large, heavy breast on one side of the chest and a small or absent breast on the opposite side. A federal law called the Women's Health and Cancer Rights Act of 1998 mandates that both breast reconstruction after mastectomy *and* surgery on the opposite breast for the purpose of achieving symmetry be covered by insurance companies.

Breast reduction surgery can be performed on a patient who has undergone radiation therapy to the breast area. It will still be possible for the patient to be checked for breast cancer and to undergo mammograms. If a breast cancer patient has large breasts and wishes to undergo breast reduction, it might be possible for her to have breast cancer removal (lumpectomy) in combination with bilateral breast reduction before the radiotherapy is given. If breast reduction is to be performed after radiotherapy, at least six months should pass between the last radiation treatment and the breast reduction surgery in order to minimize the chances for healing complications. The reduction of an irradiated breast may also have to be less aggressive to reduce the incidence of complications. The risk of some degree of breast asymmetry after all treatment is complete is significantly increased, since radiation tends to cause an unpredictable amount of breast shrinkage and nipple elevation.

REPEAT BREAST REDUCTION

A woman may need repeat breast reduction surgery for several reasons. She may have persistent symptoms after an inadequate initial reduction, or she may have recurrent symptoms because her breasts continued to enlarge. The appearance of her breasts may be unsatisfactory, or she may have significant breast asymmetry. Repeat breast reduction can be done safely, but it is extremely important that the surgeon doing the second surgery try to use the same nipple pedicle that was used the first time. The pedicle contains the blood supply to the nipple, and damage to the original pedicle compromises nipple survival. Some women undergoing repeat breast reduction will need free nipple grafts in order to assure nipple survival. I recommend that any patient considering having any kind of secondary breast reduction surgery make every effort to obtain the official operative report of the first surgery. If not too many years have passed, these reports can be obtained from the original surgeon's office or from the facility where the surgery was performed.

MASTOPEXY

Mastopexy is the technical term for breast lift. Some women do not want to have smaller breasts but want their breasts to look more youthful. Gravity and skin stretching eventually affect all breasts, and mastopexy is designed to help offset these changes. Sagging of the breasts is called ptosis, and this word actually refers to the position of the nipple in relation to the crease under the breast. In the "ideal" breast, the nipple should be slightly above the level of the breast crease (also known as the inframammary fold). In ptosis the nipple position is at or below the crease. Ptosis is categorized by its degree of severity, and in the most severe form the nipple is at the very lowest point of the breast and usually points toward the floor. Some women may have nipples that are in the "ideal" position, but most of their breast tissue has dropped lower, or "bottomed out." This condition is called pseudoptosis. Finally, there is an uncommon condition in which the crease under the breast is too high because the breast tissue in the lower portion of the breast is deficient. This is called a tubular breast deformity. A tubular breast is a congenital developmental condition, which means that it arises during adolescence and is not the result of aging, pregnancy, or other hormonal causes. Tubular breasts are abnormally narrow at the base. A woman may have a tubular deformity of one or both breasts, and if only one breast is tubular, there is usually a significant size and shape discrepancy between the two breasts.

The treatment of breast ptosis will depend on the degree of sagging, and if a woman is interested in having somewhat larger breasts, the surgeon may suggest implants. The skin incisions are limited as much as possible, and if implants are not used the breast tissue usually is manipulated and sutured to itself and to surrounding chest tissues in an attempt to improve breast shape and reduce future sagging. Mastopexy procedures can be similar to breast reduction procedures, especially for larger breasts. The correction of a tubular breast deformity is more challenging and usually requires additional manipulation.

By definition most mastopexy patients are motivated to have surgery for mainly cosmetic reasons and have few if any symptoms related to breast weight. Minimal breast weight is removed during a mastopexy, and as a rule insurance companies do not pay for this operation. A rare exception to this rule may be in the case of a tubular breast deformity, which some insurance companies may pay to have corrected, especially for a younger patient.

SPOUSES AND PARTNERS

The man in your life may have many of the same concerns and questions about breast reduction surgery that you do. He may worry about your ability to breastfeed in the future or about how your breasts will look. After surgery you will have sore breasts and scars. Your partner may have difficulty coping with your breast changes and may even suffer from impotence. The best medicine for these problems is tenderness, communication, and understanding. Most problems of this nature resolve over time. In the end, remember that these problems are not your fault.

I have had many patients comment that their husbands have been "wonderful" after surgery, helping them with dressing changes and accompanying them to every office visit. Not all partners are able to cope with the "nursing" chores after surgery. Some cannot stand the sight of blood; others are repelled by the bruising and distortion of the breasts in the early postoperative period. Still others simply do not have the patience or empathy to help someone, even a family member, through the stress of surgery and recovery.

Breasts are strong sexual symbols, especially in our society, so it is not surprising that some couples will experience sexual dysfunction after surgery. A man may be put off by his partner's breast incisions. He may view them as representing illness or may fear that touching them may cause her pain. He may have an even stronger reaction to the scars or to the distortion of the breast shape, seeing these changes as representing violence and mutilation. He may view the changes as sexual disfigurement. Fortunately, most of these reactions are temporary, and most sexual relationships return to their preoperative status in time. Problems that persist beyond six months may require counseling.

Chapter 12

Frequently Asked Questions Regarding Breast Reduction Surgery

BEFORE SURGERY

Timing

I'm getting married this summer and we hope to start a family right away. Should I wait to have a breast reduction?

It is often more difficult for a younger woman to decide when to have breast reduction surgery. I encourage you to assess your symptoms and, since they may not get better, decide how long you can live with them. If your symptoms are severe and are restricting your ability to do the things that you want to do, you should think seriously about having surgery sooner rather than later. If, on the other hand, your symptoms are annoying but intermittent and tolerable, you will have a more stable and perhaps a more aesthetically desirable result if you wait until after you finish your pregnancies.

If you decide to have surgery soon, allow yourself a minimum of two and, preferably, four to six months to heal well and to develop a better shape before your wedding and honeymoon.

My current insurance company approved the surgery and the operation is two weeks from now, but I just got a new job that starts in a month. What should I do?

First of all, you need to be sure that your current insurance policy will be in effect on your surgery date. Second, if you will be changing insurance companies after surgery, make some calls to find out if the new company will pay for any care beyond the expected routine care (such as more surgery) that you might require after the operation.

As far as your new job is concerned, you should be able to perform a desk job two weeks after surgery. Check to see if the new job has more strenuous requirements.

My surgery is next week, but we just accepted an offer on our house and have to move out in a month. Should I cancel my surgery?

You cannot be physically responsible for packing, unpacking, or moving furniture during the first month after your surgery and still expect your breasts to heal uneventfully. In a situation like this, you must understand your limitations and plan appropriately. In general, it is better to err on the side of arranging for too much help.

Insurance

My health insurance doesn't cover breast reduction surgery, but I am so lopsided after my mastectomy and reconstruction. What are my options?

The Women's Health and Cancer Rights Act of 1998 (WHCRA) is a federal law that provides protections to patients who choose to have breast reconstruction in connection with a mastectomy. This law applies generally both to women covered under group health plans and women with individual health insurance coverage. If a group health plan or health insurance issuer chooses to cover mastectomies, then the plan or issuer is generally subject to WHCRA requirements. If WHCRA applies to your case, and if you are receiving benefits in connection with a mastectomy and you elect breast reconstruction, coverage must be provided for, among other things, reconstruction of the breast on which the mastectomy has been performed *and surgery and reconstruction of the opposite breast to produce a symmetrical appearance.* Whether WHCRA or a state law that affords you the same protection as WHCRA applies to your coverage will depend on your situation. Generally, WHCRA applies if you are in a self-insured plan. Your state law will determine whether WHCRA will apply to coverage under an insured group plan, or to individual health insurance coverage. Contact your state's insurance department to find out about whether WHCRA applies to your coverage if you are *not* in a self-insured health plan.

How do I figure out how much I will have to pay after my insurance company pays its portion?

Your insurance contract will spell out its obligations and your potential financial liability. In brief, you need to know (1) if your surgery is covered; (2) if your surgeon and the facility (the providers of service) can bill you for the difference between the charges and what the insurance company approves; (3) what your co-pays are (this is usually a percentage of the approved amount, not the charged amount); and (4) what your deductible is and how much of it remains to be met. If you undergo your surgery at the end of the benefit year in which you have already had medical expenses, you may have already met the deductible, but you will still have to pay any co-pays. You can find out from your insurance company what the approved amount will be for the surgery and whether the providers of services are permitted by their contracts with the insurer to balance-bill you. If they can balance-bill, you will need to find out the providers' actual charges. If you need to know all of these numbers ahead of time, read Chapter 5 under the section Self Pay, so that you know what types of charges you can expect.

My insurance company approved my surgery but said that the surgeon has to remove at least 500 grams. What happens if the surgeon doesn't remove that amount?

Insurance companies almost always have a formula that determines the minimum weight that they require to be removed from each breast in order for the insurer to deem breast reduction surgery medically necessary (see Chapter 5). If you are a small person and the formula that your company uses does not take into account your height and build, you and your surgeon are in the difficult position of deciding whether to take the financial risk of going ahead with surgery even though the surgeon may be unable to remove the minimum weight. He or she needs to make a realistic estimate of the weight that can be removed and must not overestimate simply in order to get insurance preapproval. You need to decide if you are willing to take the risk that you will have to pay for surgery if coverage is denied after the fact for failure to meet the conditions of the preapproval. If your surgeon is concerned about reimbursement, you will probably have to sign financial-liability forms. Two things that you do not want the surgeon to do are (1) to compromise the safety or the aesthetics of the operation by taking too much tissue off merely to fulfill insurance criteria, and (2) to state an inaccurate weight in the record of your surgery, which could trigger a fraud investigation. Not all insurance companies ask for a copy of the operative and pathology reports before paying the claim, but you have to be prepared for the possibility that yours will be requested.

My insurance company won't pay for my surgery because they said I was overweight. I worked hard and lost thirty pounds, but I still weigh more than they say I should in order to qualify. My bra size went from a 44 to a 42, but I still wear a FF cup. I still have the back pain and headaches as often as I did before. What should I do?

It is now well documented that weight loss does not effectively treat breast enlargement, but some insurance companies still have strict body-weight criteria for potential breast reduction patients. I recommend that a woman who fails to meet criteria the first time around find out why she failed and address those issues. In my opinion, a thirty-pound weight loss is a good-faith effort. Since the weight loss has not helped the symptoms related to your breast size, I recommend that your efforts be documented by your plastic surgeon and that a new letter be sent to the insurance company asking for a new review of your request. There is a real possibility that surgery will be approved with the second review, assuming that you meet all other requirements.

Testing

I just had lab work done by my family doctor. Do I have to get more testing for surgery?

> Breast reduction patients are usually required to undergo only basic testing before surgery. The surgical facility probably requires that the testing be performed within a certain time period before surgery. Ask your family doctor to send your test results to the surgeon's office, and then ask the surgeon if you need to undergo further testing.

Why do I need a mammogram and what does it involve?

> If you are planning to have breast reduction surgery, your doctor may require you to have a breast X-ray (mammogram) before surgery. If you are under forty, this may be your first mammogram. Why do you need a mammogram before surgery if you are under forty? Breast reduction surgery creates significant injury to breast tissue, and those injuries heal by forming scar inside the breast. This scar tissue distorts the remaining breast tissue and creates significant changes in how the breast looks on an X-ray. Since breast cancer is a concern for all women and a mammogram is the best test currently available to diagnose breast cancer, it is important to establish on a mammogram what findings were present before breast reduction surgery. Your mammogram after surgery will document changes that are related to the surgery itself.
>
> A mammogram is performed with a special machine that is designed to X-ray the breasts using a very low dose of radiation. In order for the breast tissue to be "seen" well using a low dose of radiation, the breast must be compressed between two plates while the X-ray is taken. This compression is uncomfortable but fortunately lasts only a few seconds. It takes about twenty minutes to perform a routine mammogram of both breasts. You will need to undress from the waist up and will be given a patient gown to wear that opens in the front. The technologist (most of them are women) will position your breast on the plate. No one else will be in the room. The films will be developed and checked by the technolo-

gist to be sure that visualization of your breasts was adequate. Occasionally, a portion of the exam must be repeated. The X-ray will be "read" (interpreted) by a radiologist, a physician who specializes in performing and interpreting tests that create images of various body parts and systems. The interpretation of your mammogram will be sent in a report to your doctor. All mammogram facilities are now required to send your results to you within thirty days. You should be contacted within five working days if there is a problem with the mammogram.

The radiologist will look for abnormalities, such as masses and calcium deposits, on your mammogram. Breast reduction surgery can cause findings of this nature, as can many noncancerous conditions. The radiologist looks carefully for abnormalities that might represent breast cancer. Sometimes a mammogram is difficult to interpret, and it is extremely helpful for the radiologist to have the actual films from your previous examinations for comparison.

A mass may represent, for example, a cyst, a tumor (often not a cancer), or the result of an injury or infection. Depending on what the mass looks like to the radiologist, you may be asked to undergo a follow-up mammogram in a few months, aspiration (removing fluid with a needle), or biopsy (sampling with a needle or by surgery). These procedures may be performed by a radiologist or by a surgeon.

Calcifications are categorized as coarse or fine, and the arrangement of the calcium deposits can give the radiologist clues about their cause. Coarse calcifications (macrocalcifications) are usually related to aging breast arteries, old injuries, or inflammation, and are usually considered benign (not dangerous). Breast reduction surgery can cause the development of coarse calcifications up to several years after the surgery. Fine calcifications (microcalcifications) can represent benign conditions or may be a sign of cancer. Biopsy is usually recommended for fine calcifications.

A mammogram cannot diagnose breast cancer. If any suspicious area is seen on the X-ray, tissue must be removed for microscopic examination either by needle or open surgical biopsy. If a suspicious area is discovered on a preoperative mammogram, biopsy needs to be done before breast reduction surgery so that, should a cancer be discovered, treatment of the cancer takes priority. However, keep in mind the following statistics (2003): only one or two mammograms out of every thousand lead to a diagnosis of cancer. About 10 percent of women undergoing mammograms will require more tests, and only 8 percent to 10 percent of those women will need a biopsy. Of those biopsies, 80 percent will not show cancer.

The American Cancer Society (ACS) recommends that women utilize mammograms, clinical breast examination, and breast self-examination to maximize their chances for early detection of breast cancer. The ACS makes the following recommendations in order to assure that you get a good-quality mammogram:

- Ask to see the FDA certificate that is issued to all facilities that meet high professional standards of safety and quality.
- Use a facility that either specializes in mammograms or does many mammograms a day.
- If you are satisfied that the facility is of high quality, continue to go there on a regular basis so that your mammograms can be compared from year to year.
- Bring a list of the dates and locations of previous mammograms, biopsies, or other breast treatments.
- If you have had mammograms at another facility, you should make every attempt to get those mammograms so that they are available to the radiologist at the current examination.
- On the day of the examination, do not wear deodorant; this can interfere with the mammogram by appearing on the X-ray film as calcium spots.
- If your breasts are tender the week before your period, you should avoid mammograms during this time. The best time for you to have a mammogram is one week after your period.
- You should describe any breast symptoms or problems that you are having to the technologist performing the examination. You should be prepared to discuss any pertinent history: prior surgeries, hormone use, and family or personal history of breast cancer. You should also discuss any new findings or problems in your breasts with your doctor before scheduling a mammogram.

If you do not hear from your doctor within ten days, do not assume that your mammogram was normal—call your doctor or the facility.

SURGERY

I'm excited about the surgery but terrified of the anesthesia. I've never been put to sleep before. How can I relax about this issue?

Modern anesthesia is very safe, and anesthetic problems during breast reduction surgery are extremely rare. Even so, some women are nervous about going under anesthesia. You will meet your anesthesiologist on the morning of surgery before you go back to the operating room, and he or she can order some medication to be put into your IV that will help you relax. If you need more reassurance ahead of time, ask your surgeon's office or the facility if you can set up an interview with the anesthesiologist prior to the surgery date. Keep in mind, however, that the anesthesiologist you talk to days or weeks beforehand may not be the same one who is ultimately assigned to your surgery.

AFTER SURGERY

Healing

My surgery was a month ago but my breasts are still swollen. How long will this last?

A large part of the swelling subsides in the first few weeks, but some swelling will persist for several months. As long as you feel firmness in your breast or along the incisions, the healing process is still active and some swelling is still present. Once all of the firm areas soften, your breast size should be stable, barring significant hormone stimulation.

My breasts look "boxy" in shape. Is this normal?

Yes, but it is temporary. As the internal healing proceeds, the skin below the nipples will soften and stretch. This allows the contour of the breasts to become rounded and natural. This process takes at least four months.

I have shooting pains in my breasts, especially in the sides. How long will those last?

Some patients are more bothered by these pains than others. The pains are a normal component of the healing process and are related to irritation of the nerves and the formation of scar tissue. The pains should subside for the most part within a few weeks, but you may feel an occasional twinge for several months.

I have a small open area along the middle of my incision. There is some drainage. Should I be concerned?

Nearly everyone will have a few scabs and a small area or two that take longer to heal. This is especially common at the ends of the vertical scar where it meets the nipple and the horizontal incision. Remember that this skin was the thin, stretched skin that was originally in the upper part of your breast and now is at the point of maximum tension of your incisions. Keeping this area clean and applying antibiotic ointment will allow these areas to heal, usually in a week or two. Generally, these small areas that take longer to heal do not affect the appearance of the final scar. Another common cause of a small open area within your incision is an extruding dissolvable suture. If you see a persistent thread *after* your sutures have been removed by your surgeon, you can gently pull it out or trim it off.

I have had a hard, tender area in the middle of my right breast since surgery. When I rolled over in bed this morning, I felt something wet in my bra and found a lot of yellow drainage. How worried should I be about this and what should I do?

You probably have an area of fat necrosis (see Chapter 10), and the liquefied fat has found its way out of your breast. Most of the time, fat necrosis drains through one of the incisions. This drainage may look bad and may even smell bad, but it is good that it is coming out rather than staying in. The hard, tender area should look and feel better. If you had a fever, it will probably be gone now. Depending on how large the area of fat necrosis is inside your breast and how big the hole is through which it is draining, you will have further drainage for a few days or perhaps even a few weeks. In most cases, the point of drainage will close up once all of the dead tissue is out, and in the long run the scars frequently look no worse than they would have if there had been no prolonged drainage.

Clean your incisions as you would normally and put some extra padding into your bra. Notify your doctor's office (if you do not have a fever or any other symptoms, you can wait until normal business hours). You may be prescribed antibiotics or given new wound care instructions.

I am getting more and more bumps and redness on my breasts near the incisions. The bumps itch. What does this mean?

Bumps and redness usually represent a rash, and rashes usually mean an allergic reaction. If you have been using an over-the-counter antibiotic ointment and the rash is near your incisions, you may have developed sensitivity to the ointment. Your surgeon will probably recommend that you discontinue the ointment and may prescribe something different. Symptoms from the rash will usually subside after you stop using the ointment, but if the itching is annoying you can use topical or oral Benadryl or topical hydrocortisone cream for a few days.

It's been four months since my surgery, but I still have a hard lump under my nipple on one side. Why?

The fat in the end of the nipple pedicle often has the least robust blood supply of all tissues after breast reduction surgery and may harden during the healing process. This hardness usually goes away, but the softening process may take many months or even more than a year. It is important that you become familiar with how your breasts feel after surgery, since your family doctor may become alarmed if he or she feels the lump at your next breast examination and does not realize that it is a result of your operation.

Activity Level

I am going to stay at my mother's after surgery, but I know she'll drive me crazy after one day. How long do I need to stay there?

I recommend that breast reduction patients have someone stay with them for at least twenty-four to forty-eight hours after surgery. Patients will also need someone that they can rely on for transportation during the first week. Many patients find that doing dressing changes without assistance can be awkward. If you can manage your dressings, can arrange for someone to check on you from time to time, and do not have to be responsible for others, you can probably plan to be in your own home alone after two or three days.

My mother is going to move in with us to help with the kids, but doesn't want to be away from her home for too long. How long should I tell her that I will need her?

If you have very young children, you will need help with them for several weeks. I do not recommend heavy lifting, which includes toddlers, for four weeks after surgery, although I would venture to guess that some mothers of young children probably ignore this advice. You should be able to manage older children without help after two weeks, especially if the children are in school.

How long does my husband need to take off work after my surgery?

The answer to this depends on whether you have children and how much additional help you have lined up. The best way to be prepared is to have a frank and detailed two-way discussion with your husband ahead of time about what needs to be done and who is going to do it. Do not make any assumptions.

My incisions took about three weeks to heal, but now everything is okay. Can I go swimming? How about playing golf?

Breast reduction patients are encouraged to limit their activities after surgery for several reasons. First, excessive activity soon after surgery inevitably causes more bleeding, swelling, and pain. Second, you do not want to develop an infection through an open wound. Third, even after your skin wounds are healed your scars will not be strong for several weeks. Fourth, young scars in the skin and inside the breast are hard and tight. Until the scars start to mature and soften, you will find strenuous activity to be painful. Keeping these points in mind, you should avoid exposing your wounds to harsh (for example, heavily chlorinated) or potentially dirty water until they are healed, and you should avoid strenuous activity until your scars are strong (about four to six weeks).

My sister lives across the country and has invited me to fly out and stay with her while I am recovering. When can I go?

I recommend that patients stay close to their surgeon during the healing period, certainly until their sutures have been removed. Patients who have undergone a general anesthesia probably should also not plan to fly or drive long distances immediately after surgery because of the risk of blood clots in leg veins. I recommend that patients postpone long trips for two weeks after surgery or longer if they experience any healing delays.

We have a family wedding out of town a week after my surgery. We are going by car, but I don't have to do any of the driving. Should I plan to attend?

One week after surgery, you will probably not have a lot of energy and may not enjoy being a captive at a formal event. You will also have healing wounds and perhaps some drainage. I do not recommend that you plan to take a long car trip so soon after surgery.

Results

I'm afraid I'll be too small after surgery. What size can I expect?

Your surgeon can give you a rough guess as to your postoperative bra size, but there are no guarantees. Women who have relatively small reductions frequently wear a B or C cup after surgery. Larger patients often wear between a C and a DD cup. Your surgeon must remove the weight that is required by your insurance company and may not be able to leave you with a full C cup if you are wearing a DD now. You must also remember that all bra styles and brands fit differently. Keeping these points in mind, tell your surgeon in advance what size you would like to be, and he or she can tell you if that is a reasonable goal.

Where should I get my mammograms after surgery?

It helps the radiologist who interprets your mammograms to have access to your previous studies for comparison. I recommend that women have their mammograms at the same facility each year if possible. You can get your future mammograms wherever you have had them performed in the past.

How do I find a good bra fitter?

Look for a shop that employs certified fitters. Try the Yellow Pages in your phonebook under Brassieres or Breasts—Artificial. Alternatively, you can get a reference from organizations that assist cancer patients, such as Reach to Recovery or the American Cancer Society.

Celebration

What should I do with my old bras?

Burn them.

A Final Word

*A*s I wrote this book, I found myself wondering why we see so many women who want breast reduction surgery. Is it because we as a society are increasingly overweight? The research certainly does not support a simple link between obesity and macromastia. Is it because of chemicals and hormones in the foods that we eat and in the air that we breathe? Some people believe that environmental influences like these are causing a variety of alterations in the way our bodies develop and function. Is it because surgery has become a common and accepted way to address dissatisfaction with our bodies? Or is it simply because a woman is more likely now than ever before to make up her own mind about her future?

Even though these questions cannot be answered with certainty, I suspect each of these factors plays a role. After twenty years of talking to breast reduction patients, I sense that much of what motivates them has to do with empowerment. The women I have seen as patients have been, without exception, thinking about their futures. They know how they feel now, and they do not want to go through the rest of their lives suffering in the same way. Empowerment for these women means rejecting a life defined by chronic pain and isolation. It means taking charge and making changes in order to make their lives better. In other words, for these women empowerment means taking responsibility for their own happiness.

When you take action that results in your achieving permanent relief of pain, you regain control of your identity. Relief of pain allows you to choose the face that you want to turn toward the world each day, rather than forcing you to submit to the choice that your pain makes for you.

Women who undergo breast reduction surgery find that a whole new world opens up for them. They discover that all of the little tasks that require attention every day became easier to do, and they still have energy left over for their family and friends. Breast reduction surgery can truly be a life-changing event. It is my hope that this book has helped you to determine if breast reduction surgery is right for you.

Appendix A
Schnur Sliding Scale

Body Surface Area of Adults
Nomogram for determination of body surface area from height and weight

Height	Body surface area	Weight
cm 200 — 79 in	2.80m^2	kg 150 — 330 lb
78		145 — 320
195 — 77	2.70	140 — 310
76		135 — 300
190 — 75	2.60	130 — 290
74		125 — 280
185 — 73	2.50	270
72		120 — 260
180 — 71	2.40	115 — 250
70	2.30	110 — 240
175 — 69		105 — 230
68	2.20	100 — 220
170 — 67		
66	2.10	95 — 210
165 — 65	2.00	90 — 200
64	1.95	
160 — 63	1.90	85 — 190
62	1.85	80 — 180
155 — 61	1.80	
60	1.75	75 — 170
150 — 59	1.70	160
58	1.65	70 — 150
145 — 57	1.60	
56	1.55	65 — 140
140 — 55	1.50	130
54	1.45	60 —
135 — 53	1.40	55 — 120
52	1.35	
130 — 51	1.30	50 — 110
50	1.25	105
125 — 49	1.20	100
48	1.15	45 — 95
120 — 47	1.10	90
46		40 — 85
115 — 45	1.05	
44	1.00	80
110 — 43	0.95	35 — 75
42		70
105 — 41	1.90	kg 30 — 66 lb
40		
cm 100 — 39 in	0.86m^2	

From Schnur, P. L., et al. "Reduction Mammaplasty: Cosmetic or Reconstructive Procedure?," *Annals of Plastic Surgery*, 27: 232–237. 1991.

Body surface area (BSA) can be determined on the nomogram by drawing a line between your height and your weight. It can also be calculated by the formula:

$$BSA\ (m2) = \sqrt{([ht.\ (in.) \times wt.\ (lb.)] \div 3131)}$$

By using your BSA on the Schnur scale that follows, you can determine how much weight your surgeon must remove from each breast for you to exceed the 5th and the 22nd percentiles. One pound equals 454 grams. For an explanation of the intended use of the scale, see Chapter 5.

Body Surface Area and Cutoff Weight of Right Breast Tissue Removed

Body Surface Area (m2)	RIGHT BREAST (GM)	
	Lower 5%	Lower 22%
1.35	127	199
1.40	139	218
1.45	152	238
1.50	166	260
1.55	181	284
1.60	198	310
1.65	216	338
1.70	236	370
1.75	258	404
1.80	282	441
1.85	308	482
1.90	336	527
1.95	367	575
2.00	401	628
2.05	439	687
2.10	479	750
2.15	523	819
2.20	572	895
2.25	625	978
2.30	682	1,068
2.35	745	1,167
2.40	814	1,275
2.45	890	1,393
2.50	972	1,522
2.55	1,062	1,662

From Schnur, P. L., et al. "Reduction Mammaplasty: Cosmetic or Reconstructive Procedure?," *Annals of Plastic Surgery*, 27: 232–237, 1991.

Appendix B
How to Do Breast Self-Examination

(Adapted from the American Cancer Society Web Site, www.cancer.org)

How to Examine Your Breasts

Lie down and place your right arm behind your head. The exam is done while you are lying down, rather than standing, for the following reason: When you lie down, the breast tissue spreads evenly over your chest wall, making it much easier to feel all of the breast tissue.

Start by examining your right breast. Use the finger pads of the three middle fingers on your left hand to feel for lumps in your right breast. Use overlapping dime-sized circular motions of the finger pads to feel your breast tissue. Use three different levels of pressure to feel all of the breast tissue. Use *light* pressure to feel the tissue closest to the skin, *medium* pressure to feel a little deeper, and *firm* pressure to feel the tissue closest to the chest and ribs. A firm ridge in the lower curve of each breast is normal. If you are not sure how hard to press, talk with your doctor or nurse. Use all three levels of pressure to feel each section of the breast before moving to the next area.

Examine your entire breast in columns from top to bottom, start-ing in your armpit and moving across the breast until you reach the middle of your breastbone (sternum). Be sure to check the entire breast area in each column, starting at the top where you feel only your collarbone (clavicle) and going down until you feel only ribs. There is some evidence to suggest that the up-and-down pattern (sometimes called the vertical pattern) is the most effective way to cover the entire breast without missing any breast tissue.

Now put your left arm behind your head and perform the exam on your left breast, using the finger pads of your right hand.

Next, stand in front of a mirror with your hands pressing firmly down on your hips (this position contracts your chest muscles and helps accentuate any breast changes). Look at your breasts for any changes in size, shape, or contour, or any dimpling, redness, or scaliness of the nipple or breast skin.

Feel inside each armpit while sitting up or standing and with your arm *slightly* raised so you can examine this area thoroughly. If you raise your arm too high, you will tighten the surrounding muscles, making it harder to do a good examination.

This procedure for doing breast self-examination represents changes from previous recommendations by the American Cancer Society. These changes represent an extensive review of the medical literature along with input from an expert advisory group.

Glossary

Aesthetic surgery: Surgery performed to reshape normal structures of the body in order to improve one's appearance and self-esteem. Aesthetic surgery is usually not covered by health insurance. Also called cosmetic surgery.

Anorexia nervosa: A serious eating disorder, primarily of young women in their teens and early twenties, that is characterized by a distorted body image and a pathological fear of weight gain, leading to abnormal eating patterns, malnutrition, and dangerous weight loss.

Areola: The ring of more prominently pigmented breast skin surrounding the nipple.

Axilla: The cavity beneath the junction of the arm and shoulder girdle—i.e., armpit.

Body mass index: Body weight in kilograms divided by height in meters squared.

BRAVO study: Breast Reduction: Assessment of Value and Outcome study. This landmark study was funded by the major plastic surgery professional organizations for the purpose of documenting the medical value of breast reduction surgery. The study results were published in 2000.

Breast asymmetry: Unequal size, position, and/or shape of a woman's breasts.

Breast augmentation: Surgical enlargement of the breast, usually by insertion of an artificial implant containing saline or silicone gel.

Breast hypertrophy: Excessive breast enlargement. Also called macro-mastia or mammary hypertrophy.

Breast reduction: A surgical procedure that decreases breast size and weight while maintaining a natural breast contour and position. Also called reduction mammaplasty.

BSA: Body surface area. BSA in square meters = the square root of height in inches times weight in pounds divided by 3,131.

Bulimia: A serious eating disorder seen mainly in young women and characterized by compulsive overeating and purging (self-induced vomiting or laxative or diuretic abuse). Like anorexia nervosa, bulimia is often associated with a body image disturbance.

Carpal tunnel syndrome: Symptoms of hand numbness and weakness caused by pressure on the median nerve, a major nerve in the wrist.

Collagen: A protein that is the chief component of connective tissue (as in skin and tendons) and mature scars.

Connective tissue: The interlocking tissue that pervades, supports, and binds together other tissues and forms ligaments, tendons, and other supporting body structures.

Cosmetic surgery: See **Aesthetic surgery.**

Ectopic breast tissue: Breast tissue found outside the breast mound, such as in the armpit or associated with accessory (extra) nipples along the milk line. Microscopic breast tissue can be found almost anywhere in the chest area.

Estrogen: A variety of natural hormones that are secreted chiefly by the ovaries, placenta, fat tissue, and testes, and that stimulate the development of female secondary sex characteristics and promote the growth and maintenance of the female reproductive system. Estrogens are also manufactured for use in medications intended to mimic the physiological effect of natural estrogens.

Fat necrosis: A complication of surgery or injury in which an area of fatty tissue dies as a result of infection or insufficient blood supply.

Fibromyalgia: A poorly understood disorder seen mainly in women and characterized by pain, tenderness, and stiffness of muscles and associated connective tissue structures without inflammation or joint disease.

Free nipple grafting: A surgical procedure performed during certain breast reduction operations, wherein the nipple is completely detached from the breast at the beginning of the operation and sewn back on in a new position at the end of the procedure. Nipples managed in this manner are completely separated from their original blood and nerve supply and, like all skin grafts, survive by the ingrowth of new blood vessels at their new location.

Gastric bypass: One of several major abdominal surgeries performed for the purpose of helping the patient achieve substantial weight loss.

Gigantomastia: Massive breast enlargement due to excessive sensitivity of breast tissue to estrogen. A rare condition which usually occurs during adolescence or pregnancy.

Gynecomastia: Excessive development of the breast in a male.

Hematoma: A collection of liquid or clotted blood that forms in a tissue, organ, or body space, usually as a result of surgery or other injury.

HMO: Health Maintenance Organization. A health insurance provider that requires enrollees to use a contracted panel of physicians, hospitals, and other providers, and usually requires patients to get approval from their primary physician before seeing most specialists. HMOs have strict health care utilization rules designed to control costs. Approximately 20 percent of Americans have health insurance coverage through HMOs, although there is wide variation among the states.

Hormone Replacement Therapy (HRT): The administration of estrogen, generally to help alleviate the symptoms of menopause. The use of HRT is currently controversial.

Hypertrophic scars: Scars that are thick, red, raised, and hard, and may itch or be painful.

Implant: Any foreign material inserted into the body for medical purposes, such as silicone breast implants, artificial joints, or pacemakers.

Inferior pedicle technique: A method of breast reduction in which the blood supply to the nipple is maintained by preserving breast tissue in the central lower portion of the breast.

Inframammary crease: The crease where the lowest portion of the breast meets the chest. The underwire portion of a bra rests in this crease.

Intertrigo: Irritation of opposing skin surfaces caused by friction. Women with large breasts often develop intertrigo in the creases beneath and between their breasts. Fungal or bacterial infections may develop if the irritated area is chronically moist.

Keloids: Abnormally large scars that develop at the site of injury or surgery. In contrast to hypertrophic scars, keloids tend to enlarge rather than subside over time and may grow well beyond the boundaries of the original scar. When excised, keloids can recur in a worse form.

Lateral pedicle technique: A method of breast reduction in which the blood supply to the nipple is maintained by preservation of the lateral (toward the arm) segment of the breast.

Liposuction: A surgical technique in which body fat is removed by insertion of a hollow tube into the selected area and attaching the tube to a vacuum device. Also called suction lipectomy.

Lumpectomy: A surgical procedure in which a diseased area (such as a breast cancer) is selectively removed, allowing preservation of the rest of the body part.

Macromastia: See **Breast hypertrophy.**

Mammary hypertrophy: See **Breast hypertrophy.**

Mastectomy: Surgical removal of a breast, usually for cancer.

Mastopexy: A breast operation in which the breast mound and nipple are repositioned higher on the chest wall without removal of significant tissue weight or volume.

Medial pedicle technique: A method of breast reduction in which the blood supply to the nipple is maintained by preservation of the medial (toward the sternum, or breastbone) segment of the breast.

Menopause: The period of decreased estrogen production and natural cessation of menstruation affecting women roughly between the ages of forty-five and fifty. Menopause also occurs in younger women whose ovaries are removed or chemically suppressed.

Microcalcifications: Small calcium deposits that, when seen on a breast X-ray (mammogram), may signal breast cancer and are often an indication for a biopsy. Larger calcium deposits are called macrocalcifications and are usually not associated with a cancer.

MRI: Magnetic resonance imaging. A noninvasive diagnostic test that uses a magnet and radio waves to produce computerized images of internal body tissues.

Nerve compression syndromes: Any condition that causes symptoms, such as pain, numbness, tingling, or weakness, due to excess pressure on a nerve or nerves. Common examples are bulging spinal discs, carpal tunnel syndrome, and thoracic outlet syndrome.

Nipple pedicle: The breast tissue to which the nipple and areola are left attached during breast reduction surgery and that contains the blood and nerve supply to the nipple.

Orthopedic surgeon: A physician who specializes in a branch of medicine concerned with the correction or prevention of skeletal deformities.

Osteoporosis: A bone condition that mainly affects older women and is characterized by decrease in bone mass with decreased density and enlargement of bone spaces, producing brittleness and increased risk of fracture.

Pathological: Altered or caused by disease or illness.

Pathologist: A physician who interprets and diagnoses the changes in tissues and body fluids caused by disease, often by examining tissue under a microscope.

Periareolar technique: A method of breast surgery in which the incision and subsequent scar are confined to the circular border of the areola.

Pseudoptosis (soo doe toe' sis): A condition in which a breast mound sags lower on the chest than is ideal, but the nipple remains properly positioned in relation to the inframammary crease. Also called "bottoming out."

Ptosis (toe' sis): Generalized sagging of tissues. When a breast exhibits true ptosis, both the breast mound and the nipple have fallen below the inframammary crease. Ptosis can be the result of pregnancy, breast hypertrophy, or aging.

Puberty: The period of first becoming capable of sexual reproduction. Puberty is marked by maturation of the genital organs, development of secondary sex characteristics, and by the first occurrence of menstruation in girls, typically between the ages of eleven and fourteen.

Radiologist: A physician specializing in the use of radiant energy for diagnostic purposes and in the interpretation of X-rays and related tests.

Radiotherapy: The treatment of disease, such as cancer or abnormal scarring, by means of radiation. Also called radiation therapy.

Reconstructive surgery: Surgery performed on abnormal structures of the body, such as may be the result of congenital defects, developmental abnormalities, trauma, infection, tumors, or disease. Reconstructive surgery may be performed to improve function or to approximate a normal appearance. Reconstructive surgery is generally covered by most health insurance policies, although levels of coverage and coverage for certain procedures are policy-specific.

Reduction mammaplasty: See **Breast reduction.**

Rheumatologist: A physician who specializes in the diagnosis and treatment of a variety of diseases (such as rheumatoid arthritis) characterized by inflammation and pain in muscles or joints.

Schnur sliding scale: An assessment tool developed by Dr. Paul Schnur and used by some insurance companies to help determine which women are likely to achieve relief of symptoms after breast reduction surgery.

Scoliosis: Lateral curvature of the spine.

Seroma: A collection of clear tissue fluid, usually at the site of injury or surgery. May be the remnant of a blood collection (hematoma).

Skin necrosis: Loss of skin due to insufficient blood supply or infection.

Striae (stry' -ee): Stripes or narrow furrows in the skin, distinguished from surrounding skin by color and texture, which are due to rupture of elastic fibers and often result from skin stretching during pregnancy, weight gain, or breast hypertrophy.

Suction lipectomy (SL): See **Liposuction.**

Superior pedicle: A method of breast reduction in which the blood supply to the nipple is maintained by preservation of the superior (upper) segment of the breast.

Thoracic kyphosis: An exaggerated outward curvature of the thoracic (upper back) region of the spine.

Thoracic outlet syndrome: A nerve compression syndrome in which the brachial plexus (nerves to the arm and hand) are squeezed in a narrow space in the upper armpit where the neck, shoulder, and first rib come together.

Transsexualism: A gender identity disorder in which the affected individual desires to live as a member of the opposite sex and often chooses to undergo major "sex change" surgery in order to achieve that goal.

Tubular breast deformity: A congenital developmental breast deformity in which the breast has a narrow, constricted base from which the breast mound appears to bulge disproportionately.

Ultrasound-assisted lipoplasty (UAL): A type of liposuction in which sound waves are used to help break up tissue so that it can more easily be suctioned.

Vertical mammaplasty: A type of breast reduction design in which the final scar runs vertically from the nipple to the upper abdomen.

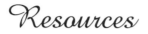
Resources

This list is by no means comprehensive, but can be used as a starting point for anyone looking for additional information or sources. Listing of retail sources does not imply endorsement of any product.

Chapter 1

Consumer Resources About Breast Reduction Surgery
- www.fda.gov/fdac/features/1997/197_brst.html
- www.plasticsurgery.org/public_education/BRAVO-Guide-to-Breast-Reduction.cfm
- www.plasticsurgery.org/public_education/procedures/Reduction-Mammaplasty.cfm

Chapter 3

Sports Bras
- www.title9sports.com
- www.activasports.com
- www.sierrablue.com

Physical therapy aids
- www.performbetter.com

Chapter 4

Physician Credentials
- American Board of Medical Specialties

1–866-ASK-ABMS (1-866-275-2267)—toll-free
www.abms.org
- American Board of Plastic Surgery
  www.abplsurg.org
- American Society of Plastic Surgeons (ASPS)
  444 E. Algonquin Rd.
  Arlington Heights, IL 60005
  www.plasticsurgery.org

  Plastic Surgeon Referral Service
  1–888–4-PLASTI (1-888-475-2784)
- American Society for Aesthetic Plastic Surgery (ASAPS)
  www.surgery.org
- Your local medical society

Surgical Facility Accreditation
- American Association for Accreditation of Ambulatory Surgery Facilities (AAAASF)
  1-888-545-5222
  www.aaaasf.org
- Accreditation Association for Ambulatory Health Care (AAAHC)
  1-847-853-6060
  www.aaahc.org
- Joint Commission on Accreditation of Healthcare Organizations (JCAHO)
  1-630-792-5005
  www.jcaho.org

Patient Safety Standards
- American Society of Plastic Surgeons
  www.plasticsurgery.org
- American College of Surgeons
  www.facs.org

Chapter 5

State Regulations of Insurance Coverage
www.nahu.org/government/charts.htm

Bibliography

Bancroft v. Tecumseh Products, U.S. District Court, E.D. Mich., Case No. 95–40466, Order Dated December 20, 1996.

Behmand, R. A., et al. Outcomes in breast reduction surgery. *Annals of Plastic Surgery*, 45:575–580, 2000.

Birtchnell, S., et al. Motivational factors in women requesting augmentation and reduction mammaplasty. *Journal of Psychosomatic Research*, 34:509–514, 1990.

Blomqvist, L., et al. Reduction mammaplasty provides long-term improvement in health status and quality of life. *Plastic and Reconstructive Surgery*, 106:991–997, 2000.

Boschert, M. T., et al. Outcome analysis of reduction mammaplasty. *Plastic and Reconstructive Surgery*, 98:451–454, 1996.

Brown, A. P., et al. Outcome of reduction mammaplasty—a patients' perspective. *British Journal of Plastic Surgery*, 53:584–587, 2000.

Brühlmann, Y., and H. Tschopp. Breast reduction improves symptoms of macromastia and has a long-lasting effect. *Annals of Plastic Surgery*, 41:240–245, 1998.

Chadbourne, E. B., et al. Clinical outcomes in reduction mammaplasty: a systematic review and meta-analysis of published studies. *Mayo Clinic Proceedings*, 76:503–510, 2001.

Chao, J. D., et al. Reduction mammaplasty is a functional operation, improving quality of life in symptomatic women: a prospective, single-center breast reduction outcome study. *Plastic and Reconstructive Surgery*, 110:1644–1654, 2002.

Collins, E. D., et al. The effectiveness of surgical and nonsurgical interventions in relieving the symptoms of macromastia. *Plastic and Reconstructive Surgery*, 109:1556–1566, 2002.

Dabbah, A., et al. Reduction mammaplasty: an outcome analysis. *Annals of Plastic Surgery*, 35:337–341, 1995.

Davis, G. M., et al. Reduction mammaplasty: longterm efficacy, morbidity, and patient satisfaction. *Plastic and Reconstructive Surgery*, 96:1106–1110, 1995.

Evans, R. D., and J. J. Ryan. Reduction mammaplasty for the teenage patient: a critical analysis. *Aesthetic Plastic Surgery*, 18:291–297, 1994.

Glatt, B., et al. A retrospective study of changes in physical symptoms and body image after reduction mammaplasty. *Plastic and Reconstructive Surgery*, 99:76–82, 1998.

Goin, J. M., and M. K. Goin. Reduction mammaplasty. *Changing the Body: Psychological Effects of Plastic Surgery*. William and Wilkins, 1981.

Goin, M. K. The psychic consequences of reduction mammaplasty. *Plastic and Reconstructive Surgery*, 59:530–534, 1977.

Goin, M. K., et al. Psychological reactions to surgery of the breast. *Plastic and Reconstructive Surgery*, 69:347–354, 1982.

Goldwyn, R. M. *Reduction Mammaplasty*. Little, Brown & Co., 1990.

Gonzalez, F., et al. Reduction mammaplasty improves symptoms of macromastia. *Plastic and Reconstructive Surgery*, 91:1270–1276, 1993.

Green, A. R. "The reason for hating myself": a patient's request for breast reduction. *British Journal of Plastic Surgery*, 49:439–441, 1996.

Harris, O. L. Self-consciousness of disproportionate breast size: a primary psychological reaction to abnormal appearance. *British Journal of Plastic Surgery*, 36:191, 1983.

Hollyman, J. A., et al. Surgery for the psyche: a longitudinal study of women undergoing reduction mammaplasty. *British Journal of Plastic Surgery*, 39:222–224, 1986.

Kerrigan, C. L., et al. Measuring health state preference in women with breast hypertrophy. *Plastic and Reconstructive Surgery*, 106:280–288, 2000.

———— Reduction mammaplasty: defining medical necessity. *Medical Decision Making*, 22:208–217, 2002.

———— The health burden of breast hypertrophy. *Plastic and Reconstructive Surgery*, 108:1591–1599, 2001.

Krieger, L. M., and M. A. Lesavoy. Managed care's methods for determining coverage of plastic surgery procedures: the example of reduction mammaplasty. *Plastic and Reconstructive Surgery*, 107:1234–1240, 2001.

Letterman, G. The effects of mammary hypertrophy on the skeletal system. *Annals of Plastic Surgery*, 5:425–431, 1980.

Losee, J. E., et al. Macromastia as an etiologic factor in bulimia nervosa. *Annals of Plastic Surgery*, 52:452–457, 2004.

———— Reduction mammaplasty in patients with bulimia nervosa. *Annals of Plastic Surgery*, 39:443–446, 1997.

McMahan, J. D., et al. Lasting success in teenage reduction mammaplasty. *Annals of Plastic Surgery*, 35:227–231, 1995.

Makki, A. S., and A. A. Ghanem. Long-term results and patient satisfaction with reduction mammaplasty. *Annals of Plastic Surgery*, 41:370–377, 1998.

Miller, A. P., et al. Breast reduction for symptomatic macromastia: can objective predictors for operative success be identified? *Plastic and Reconstructive Surgery*, 95:77–83, 1995.

Mizgala, C. L., and K. M. MacKenzie. Breast reduction outcome study. *Annals of Plastic Surgery*, 44:125–134, 2000.

Netscher, D. T., et al. Physical and psychosocial symptoms among 88 volunteer subjects compared with patients seeking plastic surgery procedures to the breast. *Plastic and Reconstructive Surgery*, 105:2366–2373, 2000.

Price, M. F., et al. Liposuction as an adjunct procedure in reduction mammaplasty. *Annals of Plastic Surgery*, 47:115–118, 2001.

Raispis, T., et al. Long-term functional results and reduction mammaplasty. *Annals of Plastic Surgery*, 34:113–116, 1995.

Schnur, P. L. Reduction mammaplasty—the Schnur sliding scale revisited. *Annals of Plastic Surgery*, 42:107–108, 1999.

Schnur, P. L., et al. Reduction mammaplasty: an outcome study. *Plastic and Reconstructive Surgery*, 100:875–883, 1997.

———— Reduction mammaplasty: cosmetic or reconstructive procedure? *Annals of Plastic Surgery*, 27:232–237, 1991.

Seitchik, M. W. Reduction mammaplasty: criteria for insurance coverage. *Plastic and Reconstructive Surgery*, 95:1029–1032, 1995.

Sommer, N. Z., et al. The prediction of breast reduction weight. *Plastic and Reconstructive Surgery*, 109:506–511, 2002.

Sood, R., et al. Effects of reduction mammaplasty on pulmonary function and symptoms of macromastia. *Plastic and Reconstructive Surgery*, 111:688–694, 2003.

Strombeck, J. O. Macromastia in women and its surgical treatment. *ACTA Chirurgica Scandinavica*, 92–103, 1964.

Tang, C. L., et al. A follow-up study of 105 women with breast cancer following reduction mammaplasty. *Plastic and Reconstructive Surgery*, 103:1687–1690, 1999.

——— Breast cancer found at the time of breast reduction. *Plastic and Reconstructive Surgery*, 103:1682–1686, 1999.

Zubowski, R., et al. Relationship of obesity and specimen weight to complications in reduction mammaplasty. *Plastic and Reconstructive Surgery*, 106:998-1003, 2000.

Index

Page numbers in *italics* refer to illustrations.